KARATE FIGHTING TECHNIQUES
The Complete Kumite

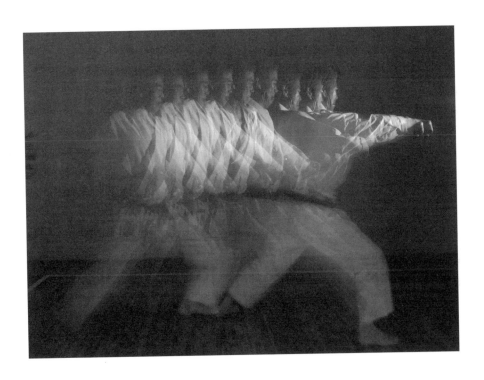

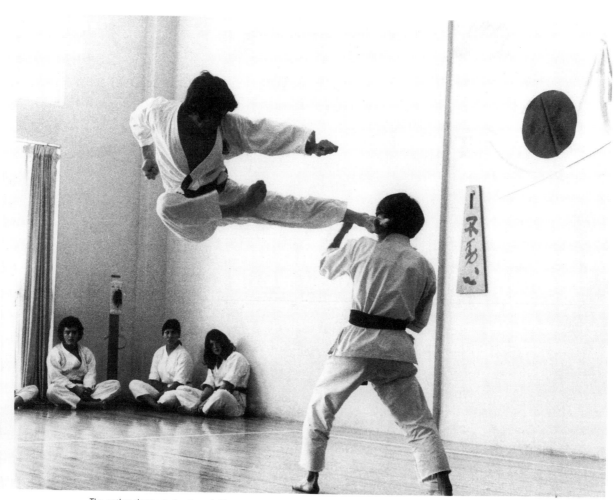

The author demonstrates to a visiting newspaper reporter the precision and control with which a kick targeting an opponent's ear can be delivered.

KARATE
FIGHTING TECHNIQUES
The Complete Kumite

Hirokazu Kanazawa

President of
Shotokan Karate-do International Federation

Translated by Richard Berger

KODANSHA INTERNATIONAL
Tokyo • New York • London

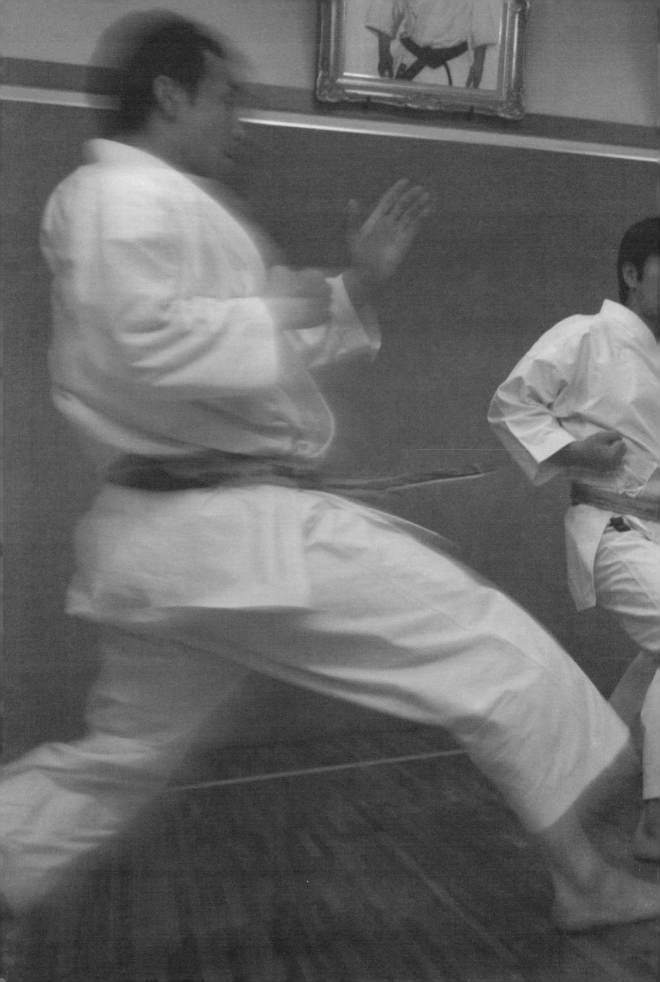

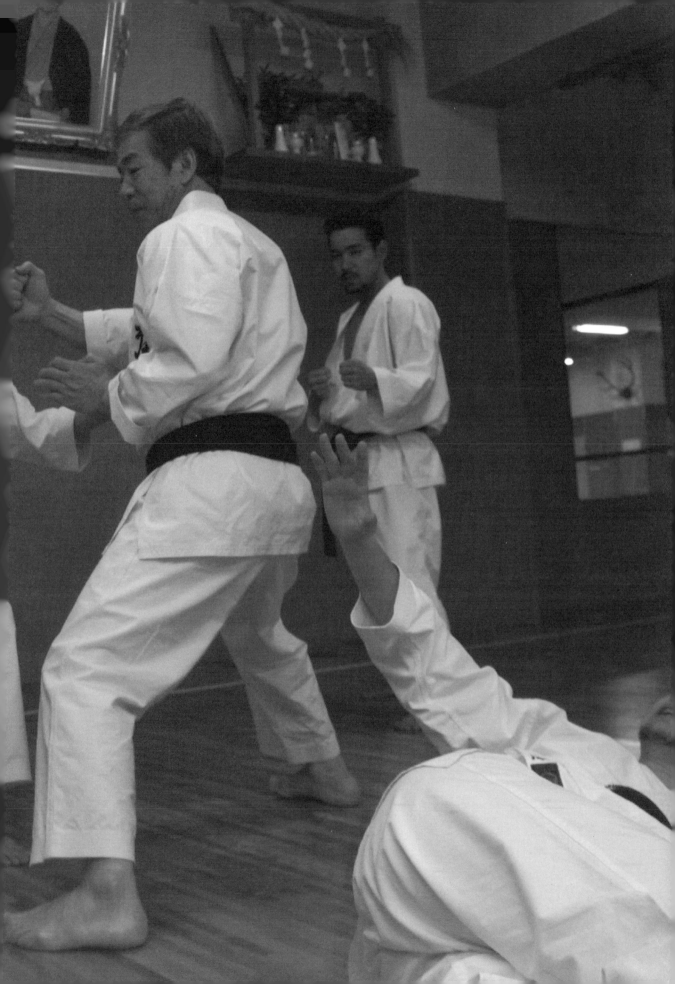

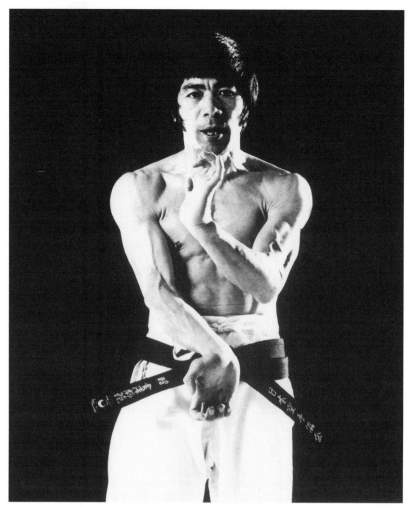

The author demonstrates proper form for a round hooking block in hourglass stance.

For information concerning the Shotokan Karate-do International Federation, please refer to the below:

2–1–20 Minami-Kugahara
Ota-ku, Tokyo
146–0084 Japan
PHONE: 81–(0)3-3754-5481   FAX: 81–(0)3-3754-5483
E-MAIL: japan@skif.jp

Jacket photos and all step-by-step photos by Naoto Suzuki.
Photos p. 1, 4–5 by Kyūzo Akashi.

Distributed in the United States by Kodansha America, Inc., 575 Lexington Avenue, New York, N.Y. 10022, and in the United Kingdom and continental Europe by Kodansha Europe Ltd., Tavern Quay, Rope Street, London SE16 7TX. Published by Kodansha International Ltd., 17-14 Otowa 1-chome, Bunkyo-ku Tokyo 112-8652, and Kodansha America, Inc.

ISBN 4-7700-2872-5

www.thejapanpage.com

CONTENTS

PRONOUNCING JAPANESE

The Japanese terms appearing in this book have been written in accordance with the modified Hepburn romanization system. With only five vowel sounds, the pronunciation of Japanese is not overly difficult once the pronunciation of each vowel has been learned.

Each vowel is pronounced as follows:

a — *ah*, as the "a" in father   o — *oh*, as the "o" in go
e — *eh*, as the "e" in get   u — *ooh*, as the "oo" in food
i — *ee*, as the "ee" in feet

Vowels with a mark above them (as in the words *jōdan* and *chūdan*) indicate lengthened vowels. They are pronounced in the same fashion as their shorter counterparts but last a little longer when spoken.

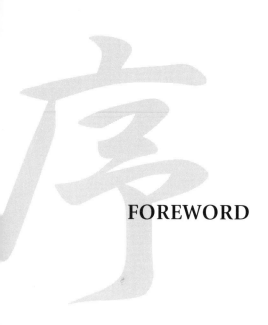

FOREWORD

In November 2002, the WKF (World Karate Federation) sponsored the 16th World Karate Championship in Madrid, Spain. The tournament attracted some 700 athletes from 82 countries and regions the world over, and featured numerous thrilling matches that often had the entire audience on their feet and cheering. Thinking back to 40 years ago, when I first headed overseas with the aim of contributing to the development of karate, I am deeply moved to see firsthand the popularity that it now enjoys.

The WKF tournament was also the first to be held in accordance with newly adopted, and greatly modified, rules. Introduced as a step toward gaining karate's inclusion in the Olympics, the new rules were ratified by the WKF congress.

While karate has spread far and wide, it has also changed considerably. When the tournament system was first introduced, techniques of lethal force were regarded as most important. Today, however, a great number of athletes attach greater importance to studying the most effective means of favorably influencing referees' decisions. In much the same way that penalties are hotly contested in soccer, the ability to compete barely within the boundaries of the rules has become an undeniable facet of sports karate.

Amidst these changes, as I write this book, I find myself reflecting on the lessons that I learned from Gichin Funakoshi, the father of modern karate. Master Funakoshi traveled to Tokyo from Okinawa in 1922 to spread karate, primarily through teaching it to university students.

I first received direct instruction from Master Funakoshi while studying at university, around the time that alumni and others were attempting to work out an adequate tournament system in preparation for the first official karate competitions. The Japan Karate Association held the 1st All-Japan Karate Championship on October 20, 1957, while the 1st All-Japan Student Karate-dō Federation Championship took place two weeks later, on November 3.

Master Funakoshi taught *yakusoku-kumite,* or promise sparring, in which the attacking technique and target are predetermined, and did not approve of the idea of karate competitions, saying: "Such a dangerous thing should not be permitted."

Shōtōkan, the world's best-known style of karate, derives its name from Funakoshi's pen name, Shōtō. It is characterized by its effective use of attacks and blocks at far *maai,* the distance maintained between opponents when sparring. Conversely, the Gōjū, Shitō and Wadō styles are acknowledged for their use of close *maai.* Additionally, each has its own unique "identity," with Gōjū recognized for its power at close distances, and Shitō its nimbleness.

The training process for karate today comprises four areas: basics (*kihon*), sparring (*kumite*), *kata* (pre-arranged series of movements and techniques), and competition. We can also divide karate into the competition-oriented "sports karate" and "*budō* (martial arts) karate," which focuses on discipline and training. Master Funakoshi, who was both an educator and a man of letters, taught the latter type of karate at universities. Additionally, if we view *kata* in terms of training on an individual, meditative level, then *kumite* represents training conducted in tandem with a partner. These contrasting elements can be compared to the two wheels of a cart.

It is a fact that, following the introduction of the tournament system, karate has spread throughout the world. Additionally, the incentive that tournaments provide for practitioners to burn their fighting spirit, or strive to become stronger, is important indeed.

This book presents a systematic approach to applied *kumite* that is designed to provide helpful information for match-style competitive *kumite.*

What is of primary importance, however, is basics (*kihon*). I developed the number system for basic *kumite* that is presented in this book soon after traveling overseas to teach karate as it provided the students with a training menu even in my absence. I recommend training in this system until the ability to react and respond becomes second nature, whether beginning from a right or left ready position.

Thorough mastery of the basics not only makes possible instantaneous reflexes during a match, it also contributes to the fostering of excellent referees. By increasing the number of skilled referees, we can dispel the apprehensions that Master Funakoshi held with regard to karate as sport. Additionally, adjustments with a partner can be made to accommodate training for people with disabilities and older practitioners.

One of the appeals of karate is that it provides an opportunity for everyone, regardless of gender or physical strength, to gain increasing confidence with each passing year.

I hope that, through a focus on the basics, this book will provide vital insight into *kumite,* whether training to discipline the mind and body, or in preparation for competition. Furthermore, I would like to request of instructors that they teach and guide their students with affection, helping them to grow into leaders in their respective fields.

As the author of this book, nothing would please me more.

LESSONS FROM THE MASTER

I first received instruction from Gichin Funakoshi while a member of the karate team at Takushoku University. I was in my twenties and Master Funakoshi was in his eighties. To my young eyes he appeared a living legend.

Now that I am in my seventies I often find myself pondering Master Funakoshi's teachings. While fondly recalling the man that he was, I would like to share some of the lessons that he imparted, along with some of my personal views on karate, which were acquired through the time I spent with Master Funakoshi.

Gichin Funakoshi was born in 1868 in Shuri, Okinawa. As he was small and weak as a child, he took lessons in karate, studying under Yasutsune Azato and Yasutsune Itosu (and, on occasion, Matsumura Sōkon). Funakoshi would attend his training sessions at night, after completing his studies for the day, and it was not unusual for him to find a new day dawning by the time he finished. He grew up to become a calligrapher and an educator, involved in the teaching of young people in his hometown.

The turning point for Funakoshi came in 1922, when he was invited to Tokyo as a representative of Okinawa Prefecture to demonstrate karate at the First Annual Athletic Exhibition, an event for young people sponsored by the Ministry of Education. The demonstration proved a great success and Funakoshi received countless requests for lessons. He decided to stay in Tokyo and remained there until his death, spreading karate as both a physical and mental discipline, primarily through teaching university students. It was this period of his life, when Funakoshi was already in his fifties, that would eventually earn him the title "The Father of Modern Karate."

At that time in Japan, people in their fifties usually lived in retirement. But Master Funakoshi resolved his calling and, despite a lack of economic support, decided to take up a new life in Tokyo. The following is a popular episode from that time.

Due to economic difficulties, Okinawa Prefecture was unable to provide Funakoshi with any financial assistance during his stay in Tokyo. As such, the Master was permitted

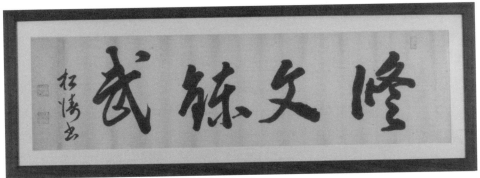

"Cultivate the literary arts, train in the military arts." Calligraphy by Master Gichin Funakoshi.

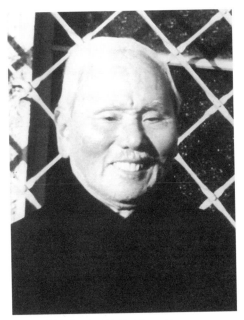

Master Gichin Funakoshi in his later years.

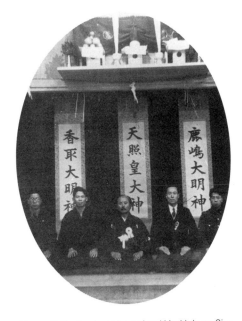

Master Gichin Funakoshi (center) and his third son, Gigo (second from left), seated beneath a Shinto altar, circa 1943.

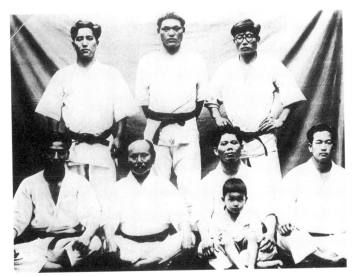

This photo was taken in 1936 at Instructor Gigo Funakoshi's home dōjō in Hongō, Tokyo. Seated in the front row from the far right are Instructor Masatoshi Nakayama, Gigo, and Master Gichin Funakoshi. Standing in the center of the back row is Instructor Motonobu Hironishi.

to live at Meisei Juku, a student dormitory for natives of Okinawa, in exchange for handling various odd jobs around the residence.

One day a reporter came to interview Funakoshi at the dormitory. When he arrived, he noticed a servant sweeping around the garden, to whom he asked in an arrogant manner: "Is Master Funakoshi around?" The servant politely ushered the man into the drawing room and requested that he wait a moment. After a short while, the servant from the garden reappeared, this time wearing more befitting attire. At that moment, the reporter realized that the servant and Master Funakoshi were one and the same. Flabbergasted, the reporter bowed deeply to Funakoshi, apologizing profusely for his earlier discourtesy. Funakoshi, however, quickly dismissed the incident and maintained a smile throughout the interview.

In his later years, Funakoshi would look back fondly on this period of his life, a time when the Master had lived in poverty. "I never considered it a hardship," he said. "Instead, thanks to my dream and aspiration to spread karate, I was quite happy."

I learned from Master Funakoshi that you can always start down a new path, regardless of your age, and that your heart determines your own happiness.

There was also an abundance of anecdotes shared among us students that came about because of our fascination at the time with the question: Is Sensei Funakoshi really strong now that he is in his eighties? One incident in particular made me realize that, despite our youth, we were no match for the Master.

I had gone to pick up Master Funakoshi and was escorting him back to our university's *dōjō* by taxi. Seated beside him and facing the front, a thought crossed my mind: What would happen now if I were to try something against Sensei Funakoshi? At that very instant, Funakoshi quietly said, "Kanazawa-san, what were you just thinking?"

"Nothing," I said in a fluster, realizing that he had read my mind. "Nothing at all."

On another occasion, I was taken by surprise when I heard Master Funakoshi admit that there were some things that he was incapable of doing.

We were practicing the *kata* Kankū-Dai. I had carefully watched Sensei Funakoshi's every move and performed each technique precisely as he had shown us. But even so, he came over to me and said, "Kanazawa-san, you should spread your feet farther apart and lower your hips more."

"Yes, sir," I said in response, but was baffled by his comment, as I had been standing just as he had shown us a moment earlier.

"I am old; I cannot do this," the Master continued. "But you are young. Youth is the time to strengthen your legs."

While practicing the same *kata*, I spread my hands in the opening move by slowly describing an arc, just as I had seen Sensei Funakoshi do. Upon seeing this, the Master said, "I do it that way because of my age. When you are young, rhythm is important." He then instructed me to perform the motion sharply, in two steps.

Youth and seasoned expertise cannot be possessed simultaneously. Since my

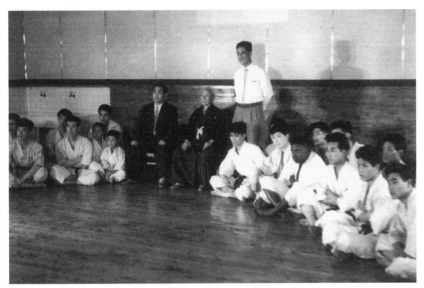

Master Gichin Funakoshi (center) watches a demonstration for the opening of the Japan Karate Association Dōjō on March 20, 1955. On either side of Funakoshi are JKA administrative director Masatomo Takagi (sitting) and Kimio Itō (standing). The author is seated on the floor in front of Itō.

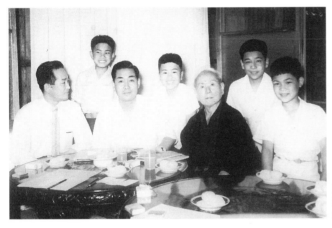

Front row, from left: Instructor Masatoshi Nakayama, Instructor Masatomo Takagi, and Master Gichin Funakoshi.

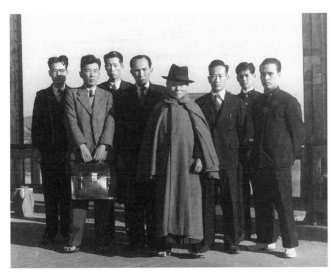

A group photo with Master Gichin Funakoshi (wearing hat). Standing on either side of Funakoshi are Mr. Obata (left) and Instructor Masatoshi Nakayama.

encounter with Master Funakoshi, the concept that one thing must be sacrificed before another can be gained has become one of my personal themes.

In the insect world, larvae and adult insects assume different appearances and have different feeding requirements. While people do not go through the same physical transformations that insects do, at each stage of human development—infancy, childhood, adolescence, adulthood, and advanced age—we are a different animal and our bodies have different requirements.

Just as Master Funakoshi used to advise against any kind of activity that inhibits flexibility during the growth phase, instructors should make a special effort to encourage infants and children to freely take part in various types of exercise. And when participating in such activities, it is important for young people to set small goals for themselves and experience the joy of achieving them. Additionally, discovering new worlds, seeing new wonders, and cultivating the mind are more important than increasing the amount of physical exercise. The heightening of sensibilities contributes not only to the future development of an intuitive martial arts sense, but also leads to the building of character.

Adolescence is a period that brings with it the turbulence and greenness of a late-spring storm. It is a time of introspection and worries, when the relationship between mind and body falls out of balance. First, feelings of inferiority, weakness, fear, and anger must be overcome through the strengthening of the self. The best means of achieving this objective is by engaging in physical exercise and becoming absorbed in it.

Master Funakoshi was fond of cleaning and I can recall his always-tidy appearance. Whenever I allowed my troubles to get the best of me, I found that exercise and cleaning enabled me to soon arrive at a solution. Even though while at university the senior students would have me scrub the dormitory hallways "until I could see what I was thinking in the floor's reflection," I believe that the foundation of karate is rooted in daily life. That is why I take special care during physical activity to equally use the left and right halves of my body, and in so doing, employ the use of all of the body's organs.

Science now shows us that balancing the use of the left and right hemispheres of the brain improves memory and that exercising the body is of prime importance. While I cannot speak from a scientific perspective, I have experienced firsthand that the appreciation and repetition of life's everyday responsibilities leads naturally to a balanced use of mind and body.

If nothing else, adolescence is a time to gain strength and build confidence. If it is not possible to like yourself, then it becomes impossible to feel compassion for others.

And the wonder drugs that link mind and body are: breathing, spirit (kiai), the abdomen, and the hips. It is these components that can take someone from the level of simply becoming stronger to achieving harmony with, and gaining control over, the self.

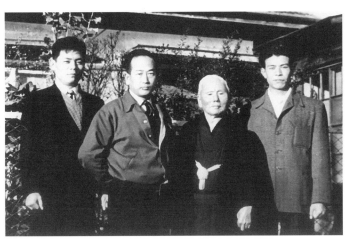

From left: Masaru Sakamoto, Instructor Masatoshi Nakayama, Master Gichin Funakoshi, and Teruyuki Okazaki.

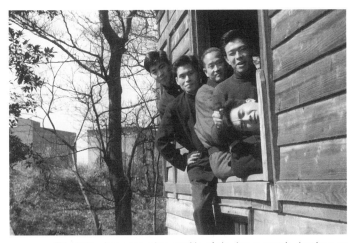

This 1954 photo was taken outside of the karate team's dormitory at Takushoku University. The author (far left), a third-year student at the time, joins his fellow team members for a snapshot with their *sempai* (senior), Masatoshi Nakayama (center). From left to right are Messrs. Mori, Nakayama, Teruyuki Okazaki (all of whom are the author's *sempai*), and Fujimoto.

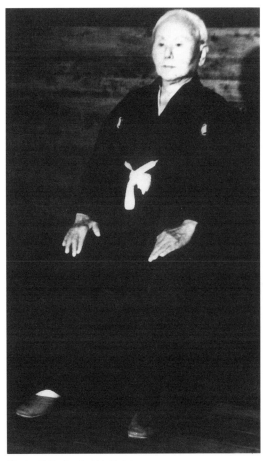

Master Gichin Funakoshi in his later years.

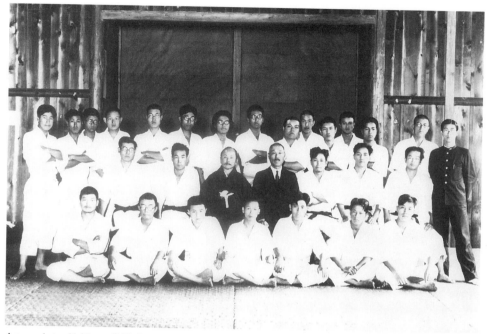

A group photo with Master Gichin Funakoshi (second row, third from left).

When I teach overseas on extended trips, even I, as an instructor, sometimes find that while I still have mental energy, my body has reached a state of exhaustion. At times like this, breathing exercises and *kiai* help me to replenish my body's energy. When I am excited, these resources enable me to suppress feelings of agitation, and when my mental energy wanes, they help me to arouse the energy from my reserves.

Once it becomes possible to achieve harmony with one's self, it is time to harmonize with others. We, as human beings, are not able to survive by ourselves. When practicing *kumite*, we must first learn to coordinate our movements with an opponent. We practice "reading" our opponent's mind, and from there we learn how to respect our opponent. Once a feeling of respect for our opponent is borne, fear disappears and we discover that we no longer have enemies.

An example from Japan's feudal times that perhaps illustrates this concept can be found in the term that was used to refer to generals of enemy armies: "honorable enemy." There is a sense of beauty in such a display of respect.

Once we learn to act in harmony with others, we move on and seek to achieve harmony with society, with nature, with the Earth, and with the universe. One of the means in which we can express this is through acknowledging others with appropriate "greetings."

In the training *dōjō*, we commonly bow three times—once to the space we share while training (the *dōjō* itself), once to our instructor(s), and once to our fellow students. Before sparring we bow once to our opponent to show respect, and when performing certain *kata* we place our hands together to signify a range of meanings—that we have no ulterior motives; the balance of yin and yang; the present that exists

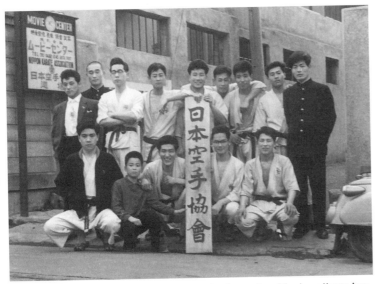

This photo was taken in 1955, not long after the opening of the Japan Karate Association Dōjō. The author (front row, far left) is wearing a JKA instructor's jacket. In the front row to the left of the signboard, on which is written Japan Karate Association, is Toshio Katō, and to the right is Satoru Iwai.

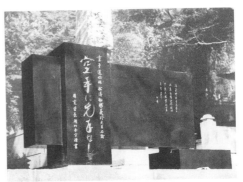

Master Gichin Funakoshi's tomb at Engaku-ji temple in Kamakura. Featured prominently on the tombstone is the second of Funakoshi's 20 guiding principles of karate—*Karate ni sen-te nashi* (There is no first strike in karate)—inscribed in the handwriting of the temple's chief priest, Sōgen Asahina.

between the past (represented by the right hand) and the future (represented by the left hand); and our reverence toward the universe. Those who fully appreciate the awe this represents take on a demeanor of dignity. And once a sense of gratitude has been acquired as a natural consequence under the supreme creator of our universe, peace of mind and a genial countenance follow.

Furthermore, there is the verbal greeting "Oss," written using the Chinese characters 押忍. The first character (押) means "push" and conveys a forward-looking attitude and fighting spirit; the second character (忍) means "endure" and conveys the idea that, through perseverance, any obstacle or setback can be overcome. The exchange of the greeting "Oss" provides us with a constant reminder that, through diligent effort and perseverance, we can achieve our goals.

What have I learned from karate? I have learned how to comport myself and how to achieve tranquility. For human beings, death is an inevitable part of life. Therefore, I would like to share what I have learned with others. To be happy while those around me are not cannot be considered true happiness. Goodwill that transcends national borders, race, and ethnicity represents the very heart of martial arts.

When I was in my twenties I first met Gichin Funakoshi, who was in his eighties, and thought to myself: I would like to be like him. And in the same way that I viewed him as an ideal for which to strive; we, too, have an obligation to live our lives to the fullest and set an example for today's youth.

That process and life itself is an art.

KUMITE

In karate, through the practice of *kata*—the prearranged forms comprising a series of offensive and defensive techniques that are performed individually against imaginary opponents—we are able to learn essential body movements and a wide array of attacks and blocks. In short, *kata* represent a veritable storehouse of diverse karate techniques.

Through *kumite*, or sparring, we learn how to employ the varied techniques that are contained within *kata* against one or more actual opponents. Accordingly, *kumite* represents the application of *kata*, and could be thought of as *kata* that requires the use of *maai* (the distance maintained between opponents during *kumite*).

In karate-dō (the way of karate), *kata* and *kumite* share equal importance, comparable to the two wheels of a cart.

Long ago, when karate was originally practiced on the island of Okinawa, the focus was mainly on *kata*, with occasional "tests of strength," called *kake-dameshi*, for *tsuki* (punching) and *uke* (blocking) techniques. It was only after Master Funakoshi introduced karate to Japan proper that an elementary form of *kumite* began to be practiced and the same level of importance was given to the training of both *kata* and *kumite*. Following many years of research, this gradually evolved into the tournament-style karate that we know today.

Kumite comprises two general categories: 1) *yakusoku kumite*, or promise sparring, in which the attacking technique and target are predetermined; and 2) *jiyū kumite*, or free sparring, in which practitioners are free to test their abilities by employing the attacking and blocking techniques of their choice.

Yakusoku-kumite can be further broken down into three sub-categories: 1) *kumite* for building strength and endurance; 2) *kumite* for learning the proper execution of techniques; and 3) *kumite* for mastering the essential components of actual combat, including timing, proper *maai*, *tenshin* (body rotation), and *tai-sabaki* (body shifting).

To elaborate further, the first sub-category, called *tanren kumite* (training *kumite*), is for building physical strength, developing physical and mental preparedness, and learning stepping techniques and proper breathing in accordance with the level of the practitioner. The second sub-category, called *kihon kumite* (basic *kumite*), emphasizes the proper execution of basic techniques and various stances. In both *tanren kumite* and *kihon kumite*, attacker and defender face each other from a set distance and alternate techniques in turn as pre-agreed. The third sub-category, called *yakusoku jiyū-kumite* (promise free sparring), approaches free sparring as there is no set distance maintained between attacker and defender, and techniques are exchanged as fast and as strongly as abilities will permit. *Yakusoku jiyū kumite* enables practitioners to study *maai*, develop a sense for sparring, and learn about such aspects as *tenshin* and *tai-sabaki*.

And lastly, representing the final stage of *kumite*, there is *jiyū kumite*, in which practitioners exchange attacks and blocks without prior consultation or warning, competing on a mental level as well as a physical level.

During *jiyū kumite*, the punches, strikes, and kicks used when attacking must be controlled, stopping a single *sun* (approx. 3 cm., or 1¼ inches) before the intended target (a practice called *sun-dome*). Making physical contact with an opponent is forbidden. Regardless of the speed and ferocity with which they may be delivered, attacking techniques must be brought to an immediate halt just before reaching the target.

Jiyū kumite can be divided into two categories: *shiai kumite* (match-style *kumite*), which presupposes actual combat; and the sports-oriented *kyōgi kumite* (tournament *kumite*).

The following chart lists the various types of *kumite* and shows how they are related:

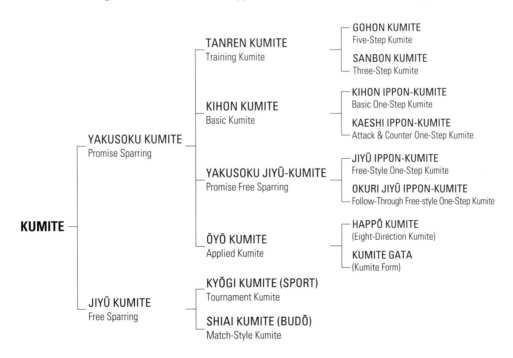

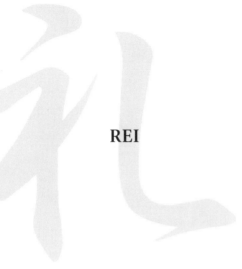

REI

What is *rei*?

Rei (bowing) is the first thing to be learned when starting down the path of karate and is an inseparable component of karate-dō. Karate-dō is a martial art and, in and of itself, has no meaning or objective. These lie in surmounting the challenges posed by the training and discipline required in learning, knowing, and following the path of karate. As Master Funakoshi wrote in his 20 principles, known as *Shōtō Nijukkun*: "Karate begins with *rei* and ends with *rei*." As such, without *rei*, there is no karate-dō.

Through *rei* we are able to show respect toward a person's character and, in doing so, establish a relationship with that person based on mutual trust, goodwill, and understanding. In society, *rei* provides us with the means of establishing a framework for interacting with others and maintaining social order. And the etiquette (*sahō*) for expressing this principle is *reigi*, or manners. Everyone who learns karate-dō must gain a deep understanding of *rei*, and must always adhere to the tenets of proper *reigi*.

The way of karate represents a presence of mind that should be applied on a daily basis. While I have presented here a rather formal explanation of the importance of *rei*, generally speaking, the term refers to the act of two people facing each other and bowing in a display of mutual trust and respect.

Rei: Proper etiquette (*Sahō*)

I would like to introduce here the proper procedure for *rei* when performing *kumite*. When the two practitioners are facing each other standing in *hachiji-dachi* (open V stance) in *shizentai* (natural posture), the attacker draws his right foot in while the defender, moving as if a mirror reflection of the attacker, draws his left foot in so that both practitioners are standing straight in *musubi-dachi* (closed V stance). Upon looking each other in the eyes, both practitioners bend forward from the waist approximately 30 degrees, keeping the upper body straight. This posture is held for approximately one second, during which time each practitioner views the vicinity immediately surrounding his opponent. Both practitioners once again stand up straight, look each other in the eyes, and resume *hachiji-dachi shizentai* (moving the same foot out that had been drawn in prior to bowing). When both attacker and defender are ready to begin, they assume their respective postures.

When training in *gohon* (five-step), *sanbon* (three-step), and *kihon ippon* (basic one-step) *kumite*, both practitioners stand at an appropriate distance from each other in *hachiji-dachi shizentai*. The attacker draws his right (or left) foot to the rear one step until he is standing in *zenkutsu-dachi* (front stance) while simultaneously performing *hidari* (or *migi*) *gedan-barai* (left [or right] downward block). The attacker then informs his opponent of the target for attack.

During this time, the defender waits while standing in *hachiji-dachi shizentai*. The attacker, by taking a step back to get into position, is displaying *reigi* to his opponent. Conversely, when training in basic techniques (which do not involve an opponent), practitioners step forward to get into position to display their fighting spirit.

After the defender has completed his counterattack, both attacker and defender once again return to *hachiji-dachi shizentai*, inhaling while returning the leg that had been moved to perform their respective techniques. Both practitioners then exhale while tightening the abdomen, concentrating the focus in the lower abdomen in preparation for the movement to follow.

Whether executing *rei*, assuming a preparatory stance, or engaging in *kumite*, breathing that is harmonious with the movement being performed and an awareness of the circumstances is of crucial importance.

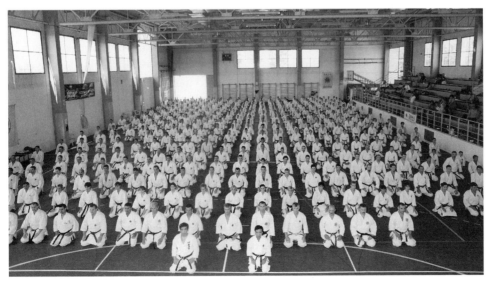

A commemorative training session in celebration of the author's 70th birthday, in the city of Igea Marina, Italy.

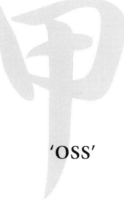

'OSS'

Within the world of Shōtōkan karate, the word "Oss" is no longer viewed in terms of its Japanese origins, but has developed into a universal greeting understood by practitioners across the globe. It is used in various situations not only for such basic everyday greetings as "hello," "goodbye," and "glad to meet you" but also to convey "thank you" and "I understand." To use "Oss" correctly, you must utter it from the lower abdomen with a properly executed bow, displaying respect, trust, and sincerity toward the person(s) to whom it is directed.

In Japanese, "Oss" is written using the Chinese characters 押忍, meaning "push" and "endure" respectively. The first character conveys a forward-looking attitude and fighting spirit, a willingness always to push forward, regardless of circumstances. The second character conveys the idea that, through perseverance, any obstacle or setback, no matter how formidable, can be overcome.

With youth comes the physical and mental strength to endure almost any hardship or challenge. Without daily training, however, these faculties will not develop. As expressed in the Japanese proverb, "A jewel will not sparkle unless polished," talents cannot be perfected without effort. The use of "Oss" as a greeting helps young people to remember this important lesson from day to day while also providing mutual encouragement to maintain the mental attitude that this lesson demands. I have heard that "Oss" was first used at Japan's naval academy.

In Japan, there have been some misunderstandings concerning "Oss," which have resulted in its use being banned in some places. I believe that this was because of some karate practitioners annoying others by repeatedly screaming, "Oss! Oss!" at tournaments and elsewhere.

"Oss" is not a word to be used casually or indiscriminately. I would like everyone who uses it to do so paying special attention to proper attitude, state of mind, and vocalization. With the chin drawn in and the back straight, "Oss" is said while bowing once. The motion, breathing, and vocalization involved contribute to the concentration of spirit and strength in the lower abdomen. Viewed in terms of the principles of Yin (negative, dark, feminine) and Yang (positive, bright, masculine), the breathing and vocalization employed in the use of "Oss" would be categorized as Yin.

Rather than do away with "Oss," I would like to encourage the understanding of this word by educating others in the value of its meaning and the proper method in which it should be used.

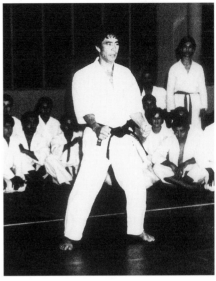

Giving instruction prior to performing a *kata*.

SAHŌ (Etiquette) FOR GOHON KUMITE (Five-Step Kumite) AND KIHON IPPON-KUMITE (Basic One-Step Kumite) (see pp. 26–27)

1. Attacker (right) and defender face off. The attacker will draw in his right foot to perform *rei* while the defender, moving as if a mirror reflection of the attacker, will draw in his left foot.

2. Both attacker and defender breathe in through the nose as they draw their feet together (the attacker moves his right foot inward, the defender his left). Both stand straight with the feeling of pushing the tops of their heads skyward.

3. Both practitioners perform *rei* while uttering "Oss," conveyed from the lower abdomen.

4. Both rise, inhaling as they straighten their posture.

5–6. Continuing to inhale, each practitioner returns the foot that had been drawn in to its original position.

7. Both exhale and tighten (focus energy in) the abdomen, and then assume a state of complete relaxation.

8. The attacker inhales while drawing back the pulling hand in preparation to perform *gedan-barai*.

9. The attacker exhales while executing *gedan-barai*, which is the starting position.

10–11. The attacker steps forward with *jōdan jun-zuki* (upper-level front punch), inhaling during the first three-quarters of the step, and finally exhaling during the final quarter step while simultaneously performing *jōdan jun-zuki*. The defender steps back with *jōdan age-uke* (upper-level rising block), breathing in during the first half of the step, and exhaling during the remaining half while simultaneously performing *jōdan age-uke*, followed by *gyaku-zuki* (reverse punch). The *gyaku-zuki* (photo 11) is performed with a short exhalation.

12–13. The attacker steps back while breathing in (extended breath). The defender, moving in synchronization with the attacker, takes a step forward while breathing in. During this motion, attention must be paid to speed, breathing, and movement. The defender must synchronize his actions to match those of the attacker.

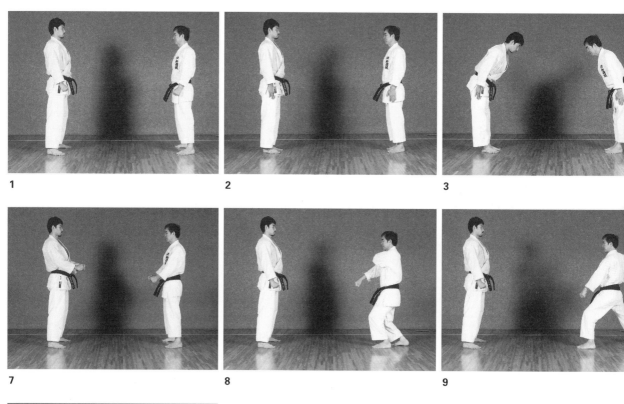

1   2   3

7   8   9

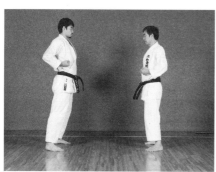

13

REI AND SAHŌ

Rei and Setsu

When interacting with others, *rei* (bowing) serves as a means of initially displaying respect for a person's character, contributes to well-balanced relationships between people, and provides a way for preserving social order. *Setsu* (principles) represent the proper etiquette for expressing this concept.

It is essential that those who practice karate maintain a deep internal understanding of *rei* and act in strict accordance to the code of *setsu*.

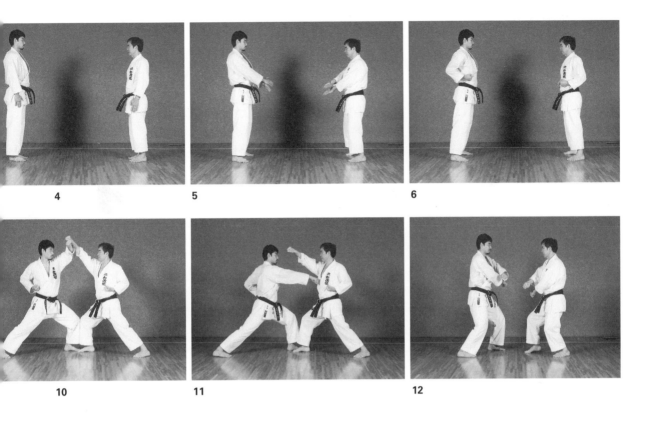

4   5   6

10   11   12

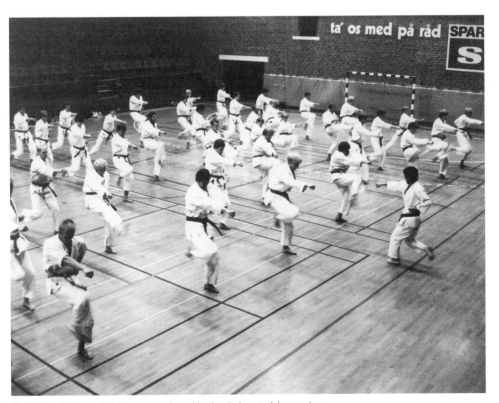

Practicing a front snap kick/reverse punch combination during a training session.

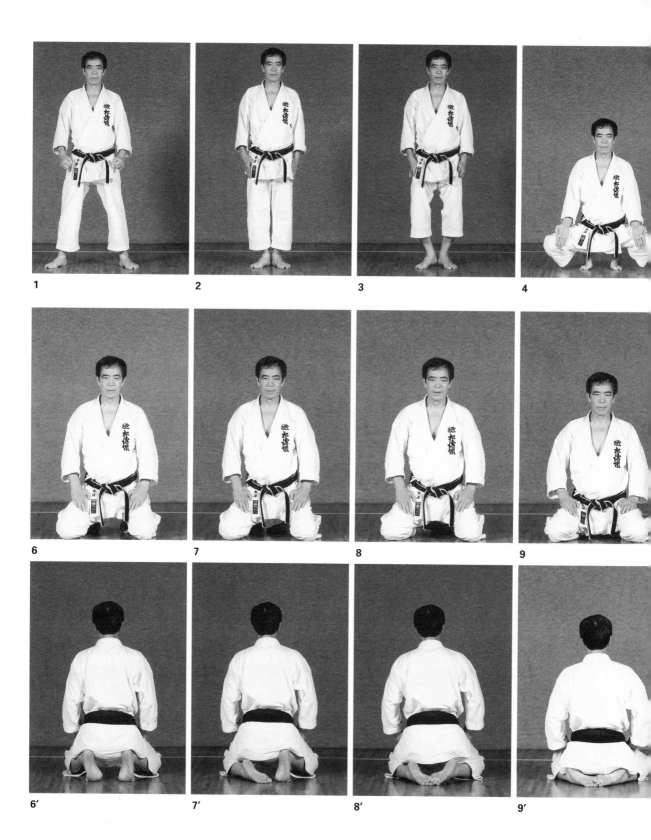

1 2 3 4

6 7 8 9

6' 7' 8' 9'

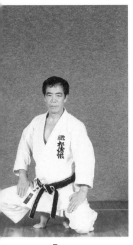

5

Sahō (Etiquette) for Kneeling (Part One)

1. *Shizentai* (Natural posture).

2–7. Inhale while assuming a squatting posture.

8–9. Quietly exhale while lowering the hips. Highly advanced practitioners (8th degree black belts and above) should rest their hands closer to their hips than their knees.

6'–9'. The squatting posture viewed from the back.

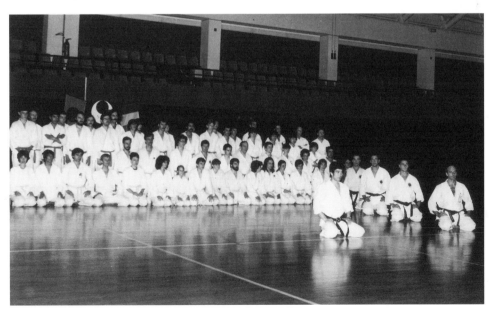

At a special class during a training camp in Italy.

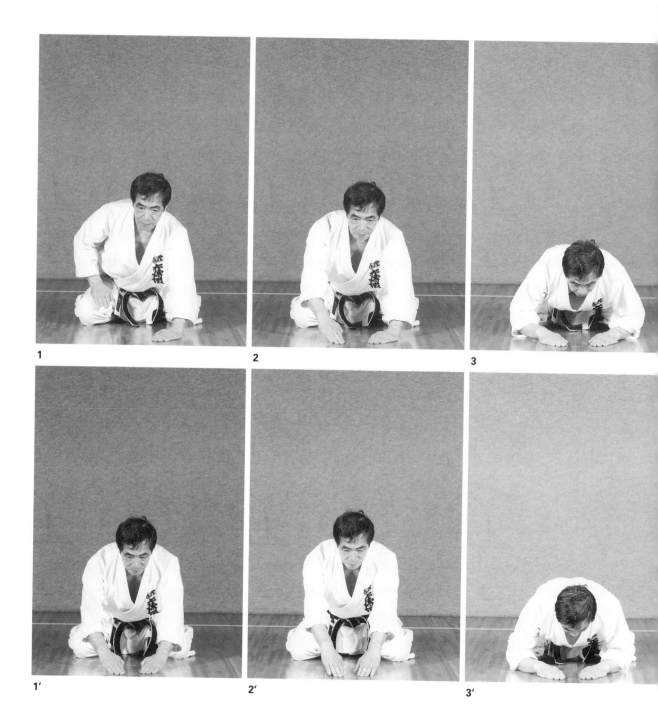

1
2
3

1'
2'
3'

Sahō for Kneeling (Part Two)

1–3. Exhale while bowing.

5. Pause for the duration of a single breath prior to standing.

6–8. Inhale while standing up.

1'–3'. Highly advanced practitioners (8th degree black belts and above) should place both hands down simultaneously.

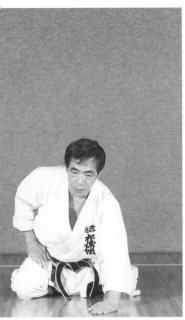

4

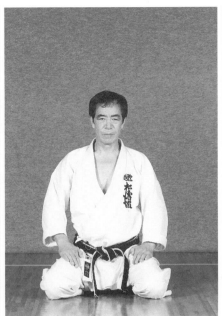

5

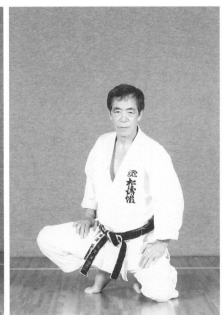

6

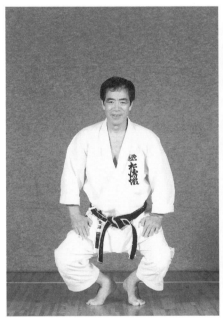

7

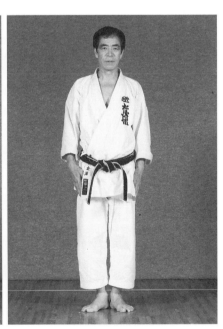

8

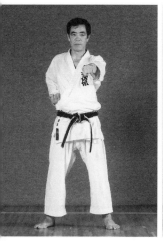
1

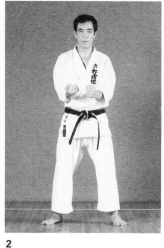
2

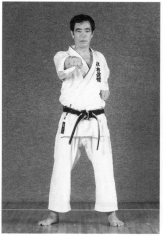
3

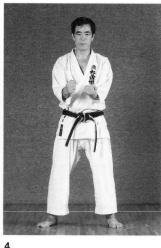
4

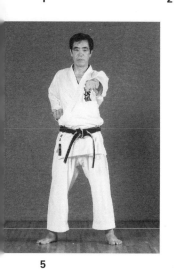
5

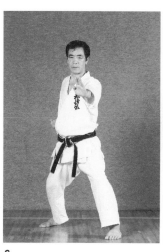
6

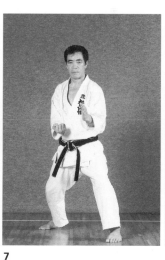
7

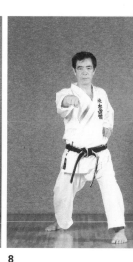
8

TSUKI

Sonoba-Zuki (Punching while Standing in Place)

1. When fully extended, the *tsuki-te* (punching hand) is not rotated.

2. At the midway point, rotate the *hiki-te* (pulling hand) halfway (90 degrees from the starting position, as in *tate-ken* [vertical-fist]). Do not rotate the *tsuki-te* (right hand in photo) until the elbow has passed the side of the body.

3. Rotate the *tsuki-te* fully 180 degrees while rotating the *hiki-te* the remaining 90 degrees.

4–5. Repeat 2 and 3 using the opposite hands.

Zenkutsu-Dachi Gyaku-Zuki (Front Stance, Reverse Punch)

6. Ready position (breathe in).

7. Hips remain at *hanmi* (45-degree angle to the front) without rotating. The fist of the *tsuki-te* (right hand in photo) does not rotate while the *hiki-te* rotates 90 degrees up to the midway point. The *tsuki-te* and the *hiki-te* move simultaneously.

8. Turn hips 45 degrees into *zenmi* (facing forward), rotate the *hiki-te* 90 degrees, and rotate the *tsuki-te* fully 180 degrees. All three of these actions are executed simultaneously using *kime* (focus). Exhale between 6 and 8.

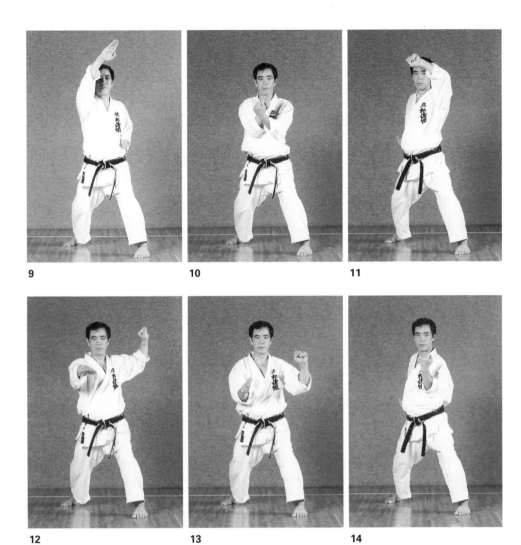

9   10   11

12   13   14

Jōdan Age-Uke (Upper-Level Rising Block)

9. Extend the *hiki-te* (right hand in photo) upward while breathing in. In this position, the wrist of the *hiki-te* should be positioned in front of the body's vertical centerline.

10. Rotate the *hiki-te* halfway up to the midway point of the technique. Do not rotate the *uke-te* (blocking hand) while raising it up to the midway point. The hips remain facing forward.

11. Turn hips 45 degrees into *hanmi* and follow through with the *uke-te* to perform *age-uke*. The actions performed in this step are executed simultaneously using *kime*. Exhale between 9 and 11.

Chūdan Soto Ude-Uke (Middle-Level Outside-to-Inside Block)

12. Ready position (breathe in).

13. Rotate the *hiki-te* (right hand in photo) halfway up to the midway point of the technique. Try not to rotate the *uke-te*. The hips remain facing forward in *zenmi*.

14. Turn hips 45 degrees into *hanmi* and follow through with the *uke-te* to perform *soto ude-uke*. The actions performed in this step are executed simultaneously using *kime*. Exhale between 12 and 14.

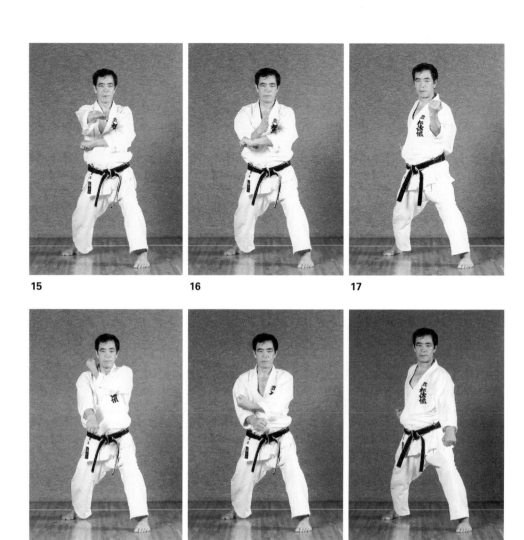

15   16   17

18   19   20

Chūdan Uchi Ude-Uke (Middle-Level Inside-to-Outside Block)

15. Ready position (breathe in).

16. Rotate the *hiki-te* (right hand in photo) halfway up to the midway point of the technique. Do not rotate the *uke-te*. The hips remain facing forward in *zenmi*.

17. Rotate the *hiki-te* the remaining 90 degrees while rotating the *uke-te* fully 180 degrees and turning the hips into *hanmi*. These three actions are executed simultaneously. Exhale between 15 and 17.

Gedan-Barai (Downward Block)

18. Ready position (breathe in).

19. Rotate the *hiki-te* (right hand in photo) halfway (90 degrees). Do not rotate the *uke-te* during the first half of the technique.

20. Rotate the *uke-te* fully while simultaneously turning the hips 45 degrees into *hanmi*. Exhale between 18 and 19.

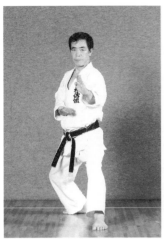 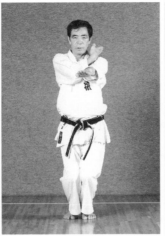 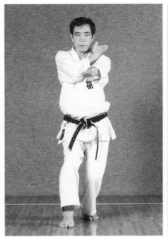 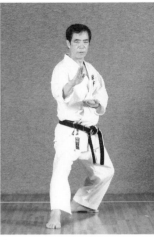

| 21 | 22 | 23 | 24 |

Chūdan Shutō-Uke (Middle-Level Knife-hand Block)

21. Ready position.

22. Draw the rear leg forward alongside of the supporting leg while simultaneously extending fully the *hiki-te* (left hand in photo). The hips face forward in *zenmi*.

23. The *hiki-te* remains extended in the ready position and the hips face forward through the first half of the step as the advancing leg moves in front of the supporting leg. Breathe in between 22 and 23.

24. During the remaining half step, exhale while simultaneously rotating both hands fully and turning the hips to perform *chūdan shutō-uke*.

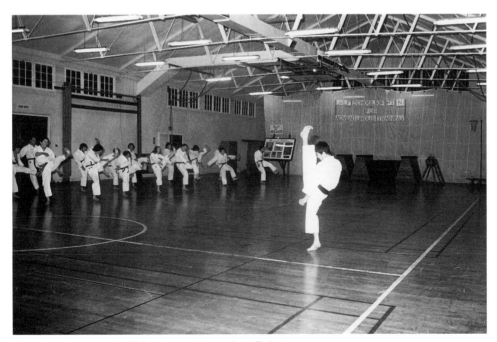

The author performs a vertical kick during a training session in England.

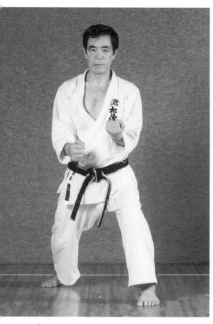

1

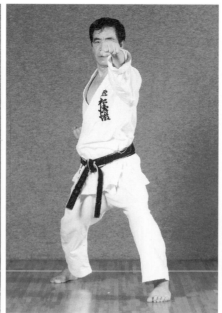

2

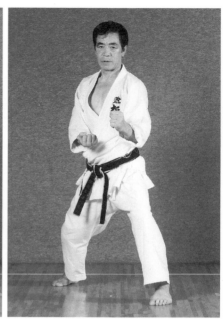

3

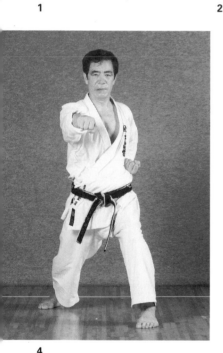

4

Tsuki (Front View)

Jōdan Jun-Zuki (Upper-Level Front Punch), Chūdan Gyaku-Zuki (Middle-Level Reverse Punch)

1–2. *Jōdan kizami-zuki* (Upper-level jab).

3–4. *Chūdan gyaku-zuki* (Middle-level reverse punch).

Jōdan Tate Shutō-Uke (Upper-Level Vertical Knife-Hand Block), Jōdan Shutō-Uchi (Upper-Level Knife-Hand Strike) (right page)

5. *Jōdan tate shutō-uke* (Upper-level vertical knife-hand block).

6. *Jōdan shutō-uchi* (Upper-level knife-hand strike) [Movements 5 and 6 are each performed with a separate exhalation in succession.]

7–9. Inhale while returning to *shizentai* (natural posture).

10. Exhale

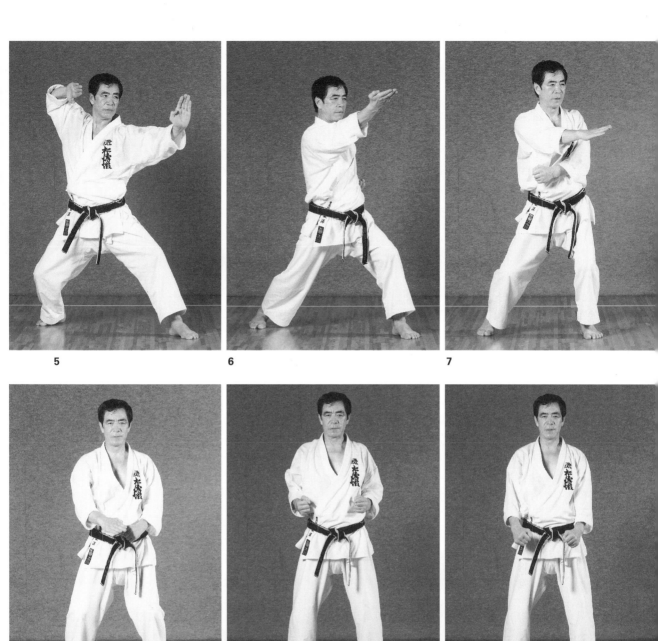

5

6

7

8

9

10

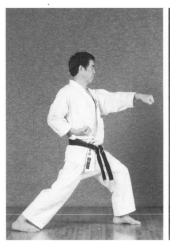 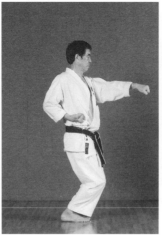 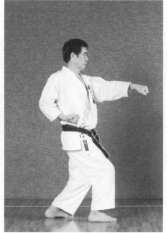 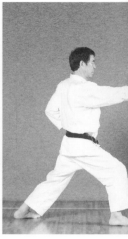

1   2   3   4

Tsuki (Side View)

Chūdan Oi-Zuki (Middle-Level Lunge Punch)

1–2. Draw the rear leg forward using the front leg. Breathe in during 1 and 2.

3–4. Execute the *tsuki* while thrusting off the foot that becomes the rear foot (left foot in photo). Continue to breathe in until 3, and exhale with *kime* during 4.

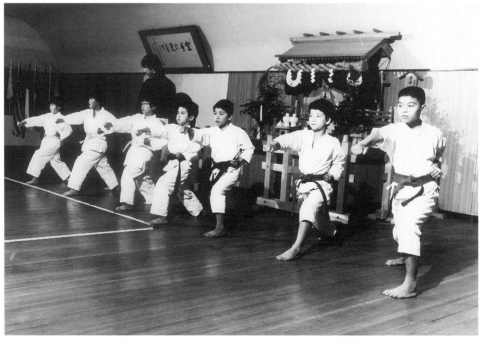

A children's class at the Japan Karate Association's former headquarters dōjō in Ebisu, Tokyo.

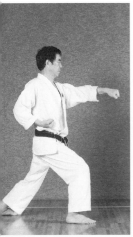 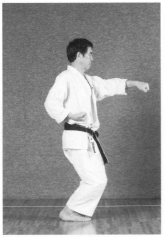 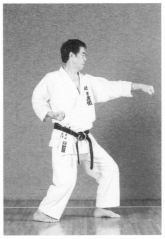 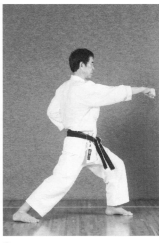

| 5 | 6 | 7 | 8 |

Chūdan Idō Gyaku-Zuki (Middle-Level Stepping Reverse Punch)

5–7. Breathe in during the first three-quarters of the step (from 5 to 7).

6–7. When stepping forward with the left foot (as shown in photos), the left fist and left hip extend forward, positioning the hips in *hanmi*.

7–8. As the left foot follows through with the remaining quarter-step, thrust off the right foot (positioning the hips in *zenmi*), while simultaneously executing *gyaku-zuki*. Exhale during 8.

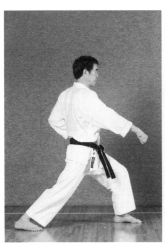 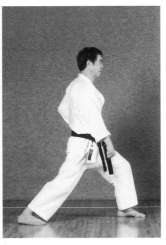 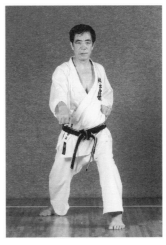

| a | b | c |

Gyaku Gedan-Barai (Reverse Downward Block)

a. Correct form.

b. Incorrect form.

c. Correct form as viewed from the front.

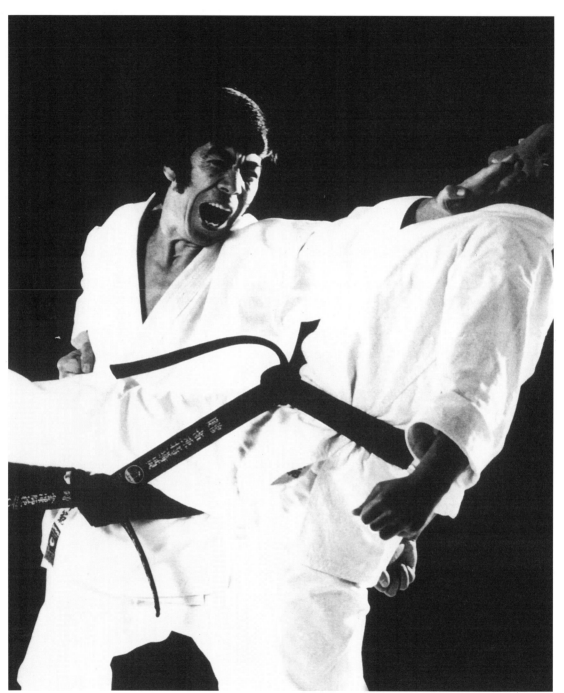

An upper-level knife-hand strike.

GOHON KUMITE (Five-Step Kumite)

Gohon kumite (five-step *kumite*) represents the basic training method for the development of physical and mental preparedness, proper breathing, and leg movement. Superlative physical strength and mental toughness are not dependent on an individual's genetic makeup; they are abilities that must be cultivated to be acquired. You could say that these attributes are determined by the amount of effort invested in developing them. Accordingly, I recommend a training method that is rational yet demanding. While training that does not involve a degree of physical fatigue makes it difficult to achieve any real improvement in physical, mental, and technical abilities, special care must be taken to ensure proper recovery following exertion.

The aim of *gohon kumite* is to develop techniques that are not only accurate but also powerful. It is practiced with a partner and involves basic punches, kicks, blocks, and stances. Despite its monotonous nature, *gohon kumite* must be practiced with utmost seriousness.

By training with a partner and paying particular attention to performing techniques accurately and as strongly as possible, *gohon kumite* facilitates the development of both physical and mental readiness. Physical readiness, or *mi-gamae*, comprises physical strength and stamina, and is marked by proper stance and posture, blocking techniques capable of handling even the strongest of attacks, and powerful hips and legs enabling the maintaining of proper balance during offensive and defensive movement. Mental readiness, or *ki-gamae*, includes such mental strengths as fighting spirit, energy, determination, fortitude, concentration, composure, and confidence.

When performing *gohon kumite*, both attacker and defender must be aware of their upper-body posture, maintaining the feeling of pushing the crown of the head upward toward the ceiling with the chin pulled back. Special effort should be made to keep the back and neck straight so that the nose and the navel are aligned vertically. This posture also applies when training in basic techniques as well as when performing *kata*.

The attacker, upon assuming the ready position, announces the target and then commences his attack, performing each successive strike not only with speed and strength but also employing proper form. Swift leg and hip movement is crucial when attacking and each of the five individual attacks must be delivered in the spirit meant by the expression "to kill with a single blow."

The defender must possess a fighting spirit that does not succumb to that of the attacker, blocking each attack fully without reacting in haste.

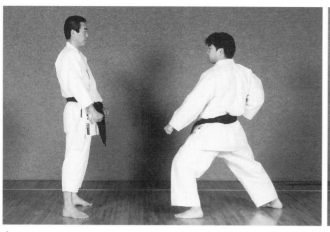

1

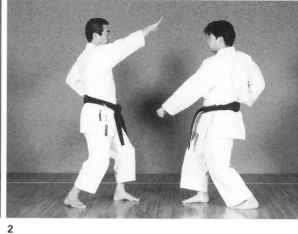

2

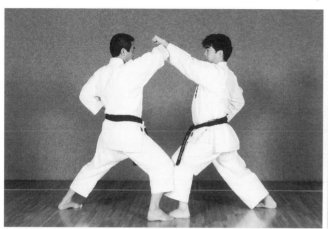

5

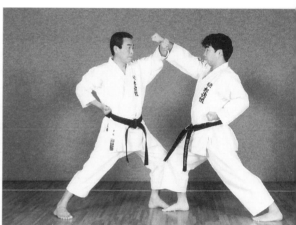

6

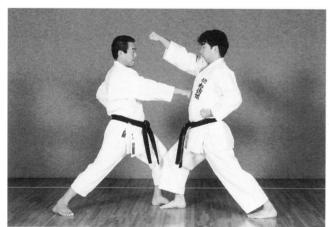

9

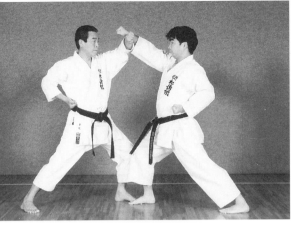

3

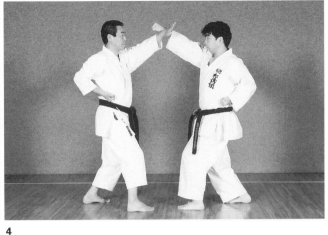

4

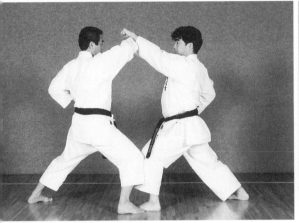

7

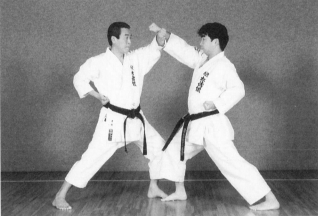

8

Jōdan (Upper-Level)

1–3. This sequence is the first of five successive stepping attacks. Breathe in between 1 and 2, and breathe out between 2 and 3.

3–5. Second stepping attack.

4. The *uke-te* (left hand in photo) opens as the defender steps back in preparation to block the next attack.

5–6. Third stepping attack.

6–7. Fourth stepping attack.

7–8. Fifth and final stepping attack.

9. *Gyaku-zuki* (reverse punch) counterattack with *kime* (focus).

From the *gedan-barai* (downward block) ready position, the attacker delivers an attack to his opponent's face as fast and as strongly as possible.

When performing successive upper-level attacks, there is a tendency for the hips to rise. Accordingly, it is necessary to attack with the feeling of lowering the hips with each successive step forward.

When defending against successive attacks, the faster the pace of the attacks, the greater the tendency to draw the hips backward in retreat. It is important to maintain confidence while stepping back, utilizing the twisting of the hips to block.

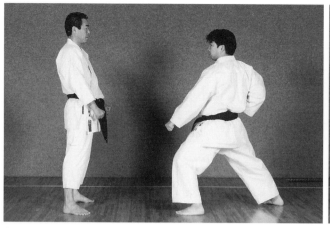

1

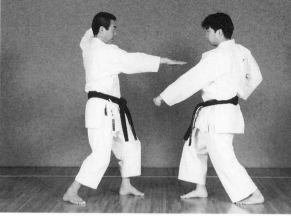

2

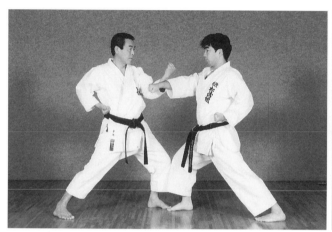

5

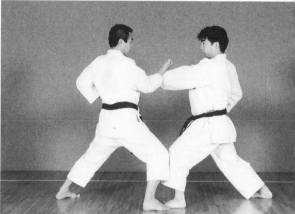

6

Chūdan (Middle-Level)

1–3. The first of five successive stepping attacks.

2–3. Rotate the *uke-te* (left hand in photo) outward fully to the side and then draw it inward for the block. The *uke-te* inscribes a large arc, twisting inward to complete the block.

3–4. Second stepping attack.

4–5. Third stepping attack.

5–6. Fourth stepping attack.

6–7. Fifth and final stepping attack.

8. *Gyaku-zuki* counterattack with *kime*.

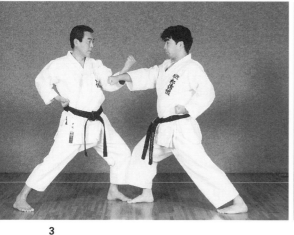

3

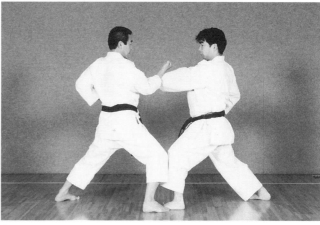

4

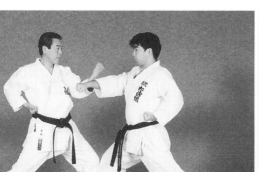

7

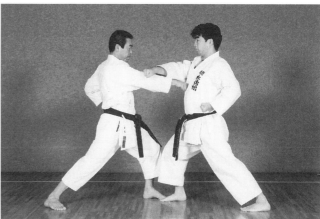

8

The attacker, aiming for the solar plexus, swiftly delivers an attack with the feeling that the *tsuki-te* (punching hand) could fully penetrate his opponent.

When performing successive middle-level attacks, there is a tendency for the upper body to lean forward. To ensure proper form, it is necessary to maintain the feeling of attacking from the lower stomach.

For the defender, it is important to utilize not just the arms but also the hips and body to block each attack. Doing so will result in a more effective and decisive counterattack following the fifth stepping attack.

SANBON KUMITE (Three-Step Kumite)

As a basic training method, *sanbon kumite* (three-step *kumite*) is identical to *gohon kumite* (five-step *kumite*) in terms of the benefits it offers with regard to the development of physical and mental preparedness, proper breathing, leg movement, and physical strength. Unlike *gohon kumite*, however, in which the target remains the same for all five consecutive attacks, *sanbon kumite* comprises different techniques and targets for each of the three successive attacks: upper-level, middle-level, and front snap kick.

For *gohon kumite*, the defender uses the same blocking technique to defend against all five attacks and then concludes with a counterattack. In contrast, *sanbon kumite* requires the defender to use a different blocking technique against each of the three different attacks and, after blocking the third attack, immediately deliver a counterattack.

While *gohon kumite* is more effective for building endurance, *sanbon kumite* is the recommended training method for developing balance during successive movements. *Sanbon kumite* should always be practiced from both the left and right sides.

The attacker, after assuming the ready position with the same level of physical and mental preparedness as in *gohon kumite*, announces the targets—*jōdan* (upper level), *chūdan*, (middle level) *mae-geri* (front snap kick)—and then launches his attack with force and precision. Concentrating energy in the lower abdomen, the attacker must maintain a balanced posture abounding with determination, generating explosive force from the lower abdomen for each individual attack.

The defender responds with a fighting spirit that does not succumb to that of the attacker. To do so, the defender must carefully read his opponent's breathing and movement.

Proper breathing is essential for both attacker and defender. For example, whether attacking or blocking, each must inhale during the first three-quarters of each step, and exhale during the final quarter step while simultaneously performing either the attacking or blocking technique.

Since *tanren* (training) *kumite*, such as *sanbon kumite* and *gohon kumite*, provides the foundation on which *jiyū kumite* (free sparring) is built, much effort needs to be made in its practice.

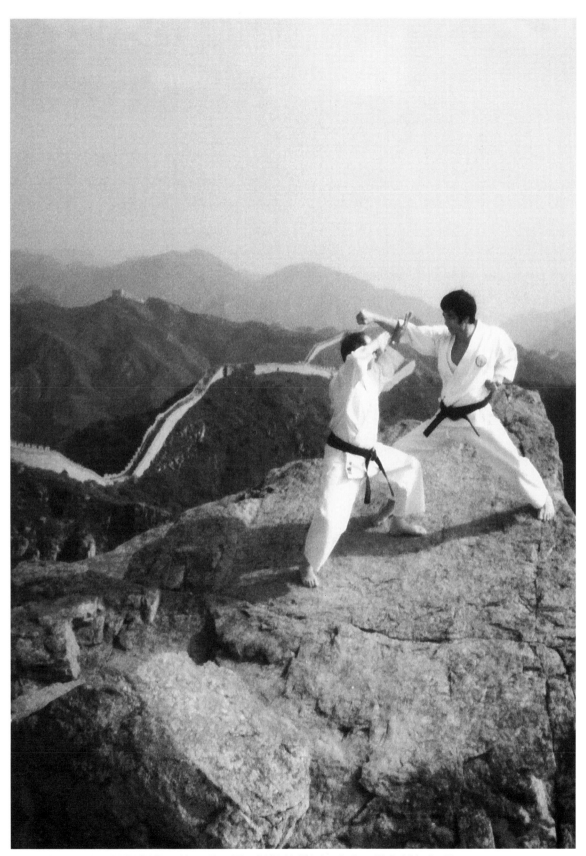

A karate demonstration with Tai Chi Chuan Master Yang Ming-Shi (Yō Meiji) before the Great Wall of China in 1981.

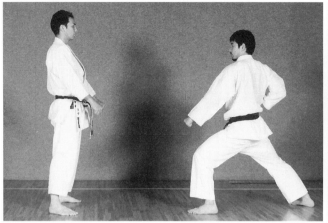

1

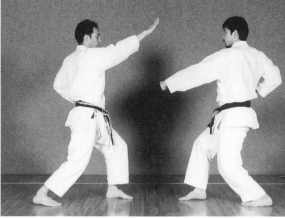

2

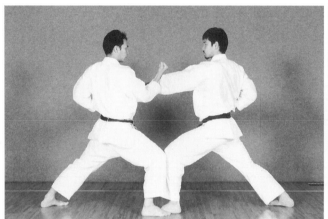

5

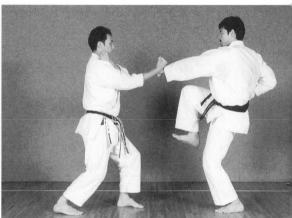

6

SANBON KUMITE NO. 1

Jōdan, Chūdan, Mae-Geri (Upper-Level, Middle-Level, Front Snap Kick)

1–3. The first of three successive attacks.

3–5. Second attack. Following the *soto ude-uke* (outside-to-inside block), the defender pulls back the hand that will be the *uke-te* (blocking hand) for the third attack (left hand in photo 6) to just above the opposite shoulder in preparation for the *gedan-barai* (downward block) that follows.

5–7. Third and final attack.

8. *Gyaku-zuki* (reverse punch) counterattack with *kime* (focus).

The attacker first informs the defender of the attacks to follow—*jōdan, chūdan, mae-geri*—and then begins his attack.

When performing successive attacks the hips should not rise and fall, they should be kept at the same height as each technique is delivered accurately to the intended target with speed and strength.

The defender must adjust his breathing to match that of the attacker's while moving. For the second block, breathe in during the first three-quarters of the step back

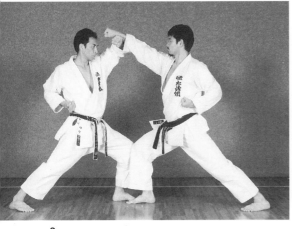

3

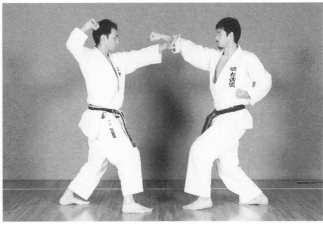

4

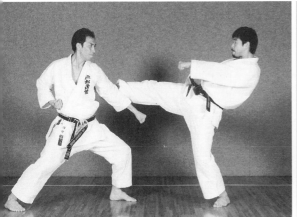

7

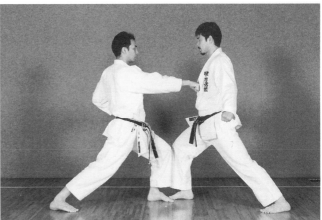

8

(photos 3 and 4) while turning the blocking arm outward. Exhale during the remaining quarter-step while rotating the blocking arm inward to execute *soto ude-uke* (photo 5). The arm and hips are rotated in unison.

When performing *gedan-barai* against the third attack, bring the *uke-te* (left hand in photo) up to just above the opposite shoulder by the time the retreating foot has completed three-quarters of the step back (photo 6). When performing this motion, the *uke-te* should travel the shortest route possible.

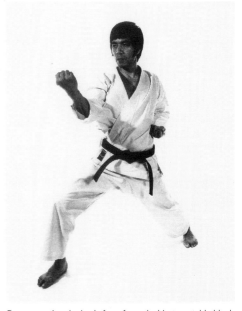

Demonstrating the basic form for an inside-to-outside block.

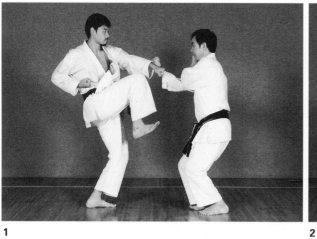

1

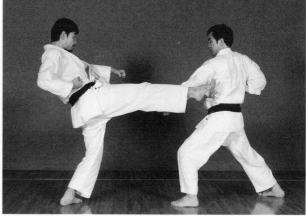

2

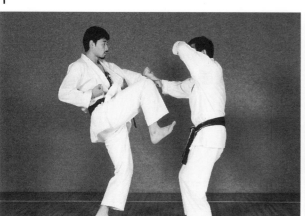

1'

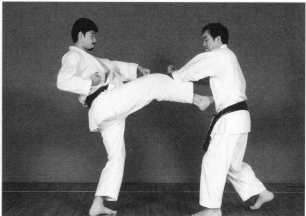

2'

1. Correct form.

2. Correct form.

1'. Incorrect form. The shoulder of the blocking arm has risen and the arm has been swung around.

2'. Incorrect form. The underarm of the blocking arm is exposed and the *uke-te* is extended too far out in front of the body.

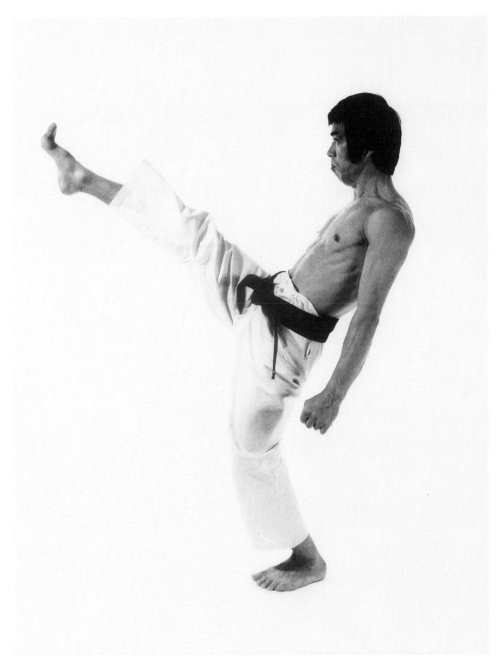

Demonstrating a front snap kick.

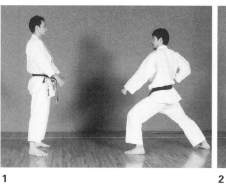
1

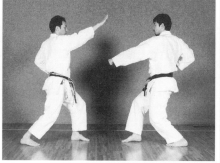
2

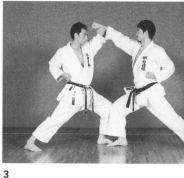
3

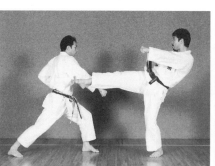
7

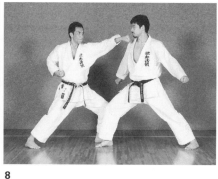
8

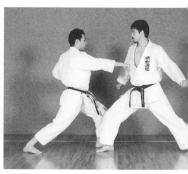
9

SANBON KUMITE NO. 2

Jōdan, Chūdan, Mae-Geri

1–3. The first of three successive attacks.

3–5. Second attack.

5–7. Third and final attack.

8–9. Continuous techniques: *Jōdan kizami-zuki* (upper-level jab) followed by *gyaku-zuki* with *kime*.

When performing *uchi ude-uke* (inside-to-outside block) against the second attack, breathe in during the first three-quarters of the step back (photos 3 and 4) while drawing the *uke-te* (right hand in photo) beneath the underarm of the opposite side. When the *uke-te* is drawn back prior to performing the block (photo 4), the back of the hand faces upward. Exhale during the remaining quarter-step while rotating the blocking arm outward to execute *uchi ude-uke* (photo 5).

Contracting the chest when breathing in and expanding it when breathing out is known as inverse breathing. Inverse breathing is used when performing *uchi ude-uke*.

When performing *gyaku gedan-barai* (reverse downward block) against the third attack, the blocking arm extends downward and to the front at a 45-degree angle. Doing so makes possible the delivery of a more effective *kizami-zuki*.

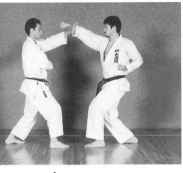

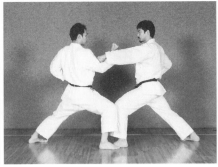

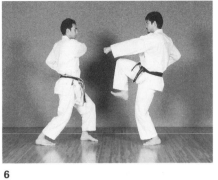

4 5 6

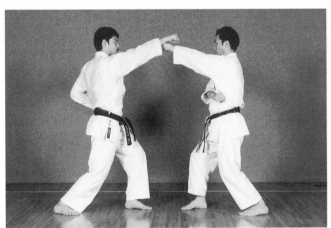

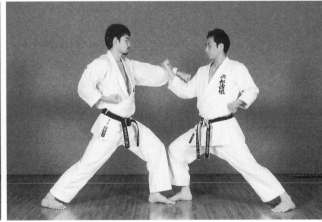

1 2

Sanbon Kumite No. 2—Supplement: Uchi Ude-Uke

1. Do not rotate the hips until the *uke-te* (right hand in photo) has been drawn to the underarm of the opposite side.

2. During the last quarter-step, rotate the hips while simultaneously executing *uchi ude-uke*.

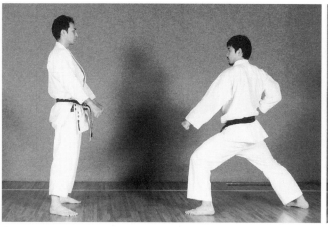

1

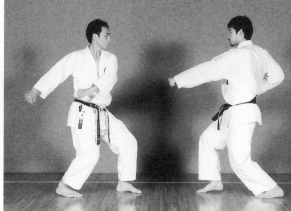

2

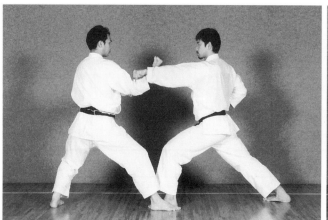

5

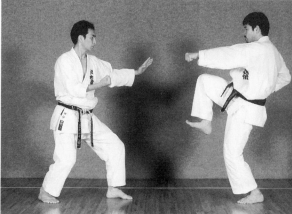

6

SANBON KUMITE NO. 3

Jōdan, Chūdan, Mae-Geri

1–3. The first of three successive attacks.

3–5. Second attack.

5–7. Third and final attack.

8. *Gyaku-zuki* counterattack with *kime*.

When performing *morote uchi ude-uke* (augmented inside-to-outside block) against the second attack (photos 4 and 5), make full use of the twisting of the hips and pull back the elbow of the arm that will be used to support the block (left arm in photo) as if executing an elbow strike to the rear (photo 3). Doing so will enable the block to be performed with greater ease.

To execute *sukui-uke* (scooping block) against the third attack, catch the attacker's kicking foot and draw him near, shifting into *kōkutsu-dachi* (back stance) (photo 7). Immediately thrust off the rear foot (right foot in photo), shifting into *zenkutsu-dachi* (front stance) while simultaneously executing *gyaku-zuki* (photo 8).

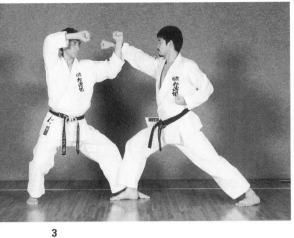

3

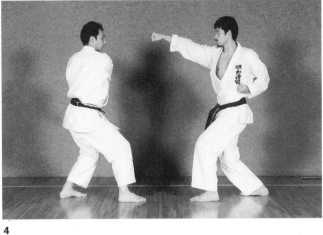

4

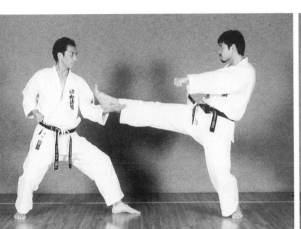

7

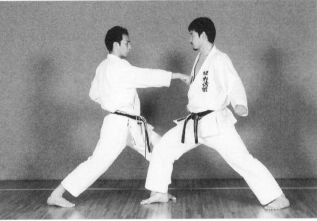

8

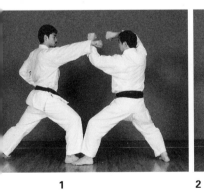

1

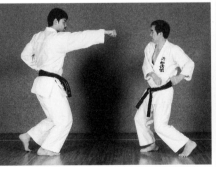

2

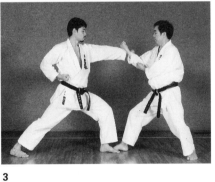

3

Sanbon Kumite No. 3—Supplement

Following the *haiwan-uke* (back-arm block) against the first attack, step back by sharply pulling back the elbow of the blocking arm (left arm in photo) and execute *morote uchi ude-uke*.

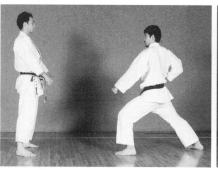
1

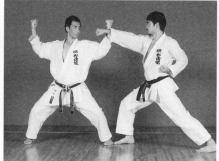
2

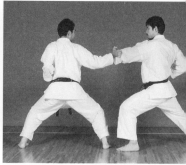
3

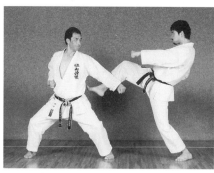
4

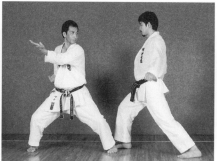
5

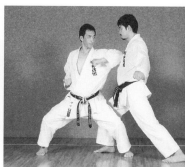
6

SANBON KUMITE NO. 4

Jōdan, Chūdan, Mae-Geri

1. Ready position.
2. *Jōdan yama-uke* (Upper-level mountain block).
3. *Chūdan teishō-uke* (Middle-level palm-heel block).
4. *Gedan-uke* (Downward block).
5–6. *Chūdan yoko empi-uchi* (Middle-level side elbow strike)
1–6. Special attention must be paid to proper form, maintaining a strong *kiba-dachi* (straddle-leg stance) throughout and keeping the underarms firmly tightened for each of the three consecutive blocks.

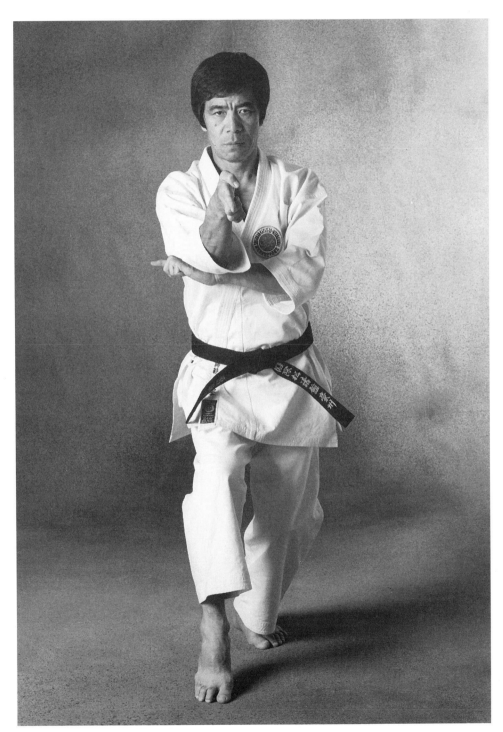

Performing a chicken-head-wrist block.

KISO KUMITE (Fundamental Kumite)

As I mentioned in the foreword, Gichin Funakoshi did not approve of karate competitions, saying, "Such a dangerous thing should not be permitted," and would not teach *jiyū kumite* (free sparring). In keeping with Master Funakoshi's wish to prevent injuries, when the tournament system was established around 1957, permission to compete was granted only to black-belt-level practitioners. The black belts, through the mastery of *kihon kumite* (basic *kumite*), had gained complete control of their techniques and were capable of bringing attacks to a halt just before making contact with intended targets.

Today, however, sparring competitions are popular not only among young boys and girls, but also among practitioners who have yet to reach the level of black belt. This is due to the lengthy amount of time required before complete control of punches and kicks can be attained. *Kiso kumite* (fundamental *kumite*), however, provides young people and pre-black-belt practitioners, who have not achieved technical proficiency, with an enjoyable and safe means of engaging in competitive sparring.

The primary objective of *kiso kumite* is the development of well-timed responses. This is achieved first by learning how to control the left and right sides, and upper (hands) and lower (legs) parts of the body, and then by training to develop the "feel" and body movements necessary for effectively coordinating one's actions to match those of an opponent.

When practicing *kiso kumite*, both participants should maintain a consistent *maai* (distance between opponents during *kumite*) at all times. The *maai* should not permit either participant's hands or feet to reach his opponent. The defender must coordinate his movements with those of the attacker to ensure that this *maai* always stays the same.

Should the attacker launch an attack stepping forward with his front or rear leg, it is important that the defender simultaneously step straight back with either his front or rear leg while blocking. When the attacker begins an attack stepping forward with his front leg, he will immediately draw his rear foot forward the same distance that his front foot traveled to quickly establish a stance from which a subsequent attack can be launched. Should the defender, in response, step back with the rear leg while blocking, he will likewise immediately draw his front foot back the same distance that his rear foot moved. The attacker will advance while attacking two times and the defender will retreat while blocking each time, after which the defender will immediately deliver a counterattack.

An important point to remember when practicing *kiso kumite* is that blocks and counterattacks must always be executed simultaneously with the movement of the legs.

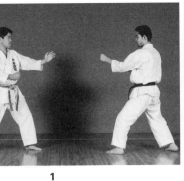
1

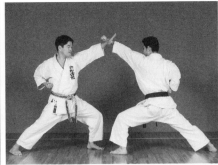
2

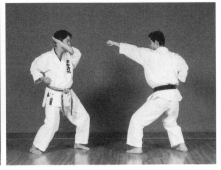
3

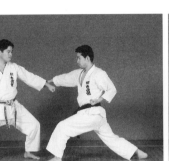
4

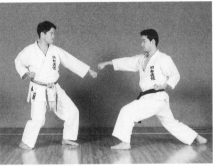
5

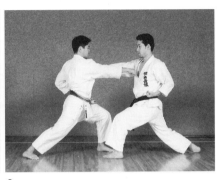
6

KISO KUMITE NO. 1

It is important to synchronize and balance movement (stepping and techniques), breathing, strength, and speed with those of one's opponent.

1–2. The attacker (right) delivers *jōdan kizami-zuki* (upper-level jab); the defender blocks with *jōdan harai-uke* (upper-level sweeping block).

As the attacker steps forward with *jōdan kizami-zuki*, the defender steps back with his rear foot (right foot in photo) and blocks with *jōdan harai-uke*.

3. As the attacker draws his rear foot one-half step forward, the defender moves his front foot one-half step back.

4. The attacker delivers *chūdan gyaku-zuki* (middle-level reverse punch); the defender blocks with *gedan barai* (downward block).

As the attacker steps forward with *chūdan gyaku-zuki*, the defender steps back with his rear foot and blocks with *gedan barai*.

5. Following the *gedan barai*, the defender draws his front foot back one-half step for a mere instant. At this moment, it is important that the hips remain at the same height.

6. After the half-step back, the defender steps forward with his front foot and executes *chūdan gyaku-zuki*.

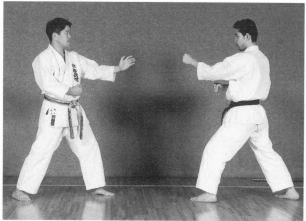

1

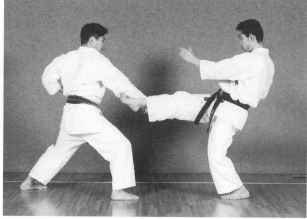

3

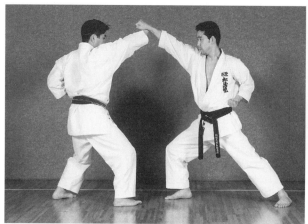

2

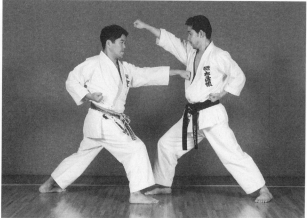

4

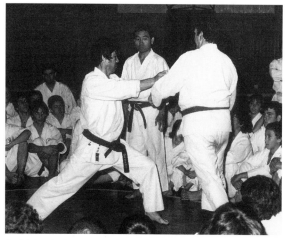

Explaining the importance of properly using the back during a training session in Lebanon.

KISO KUMITE NO. 2

1–2. The attacker (right) delivers *chūdan mae-geri* (middle-level front snap kick); the defender blocks with *gedan barai*.

As the attacker advances with *chūdan mae-geri*, the defender takes a full step back with his front foot (left foot in photo) and blocks with *gedan barai*.

3. As the attacker follows through with *jōdan oi-zuki* (upper-level lunge punch), the defender draws the front foot (right foot in photo) back one-half step and blocks with *jōdan age-uke* (upper-level rising block).

4. The defender steps forward with front leg and executes *chūdan gyaku-zuki*.

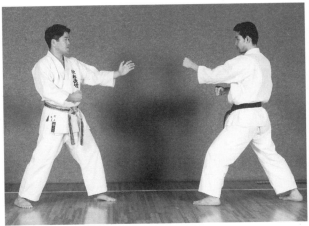

1

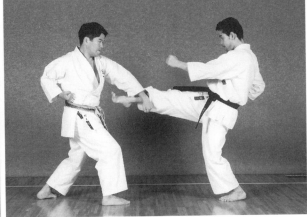

2

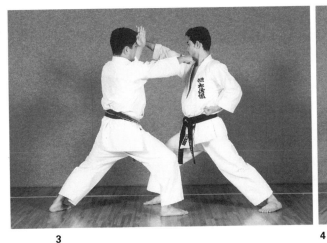

3

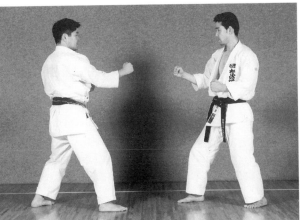

4

KISO KUMITE NO. 3

1–2. As the attacker (right) delivers *mae-geri*, the defender steps back three-quarters of a step with the front foot (left foot in photo) while blocking with *gyaku gedan-barai* (reverse downward block).

3. As the attacker follows through with *jōdan oi-zuki*, the defender steps forward with the front foot (right foot in photo), deflecting the attack with *harai-uke* (sweeping block) while simultaneously countering with *jōdan jun-zuki* (upper-level front punch).

KIHON IPPON-KUMITE (Basic One-Step Kumite)

Kihon ippon-kumite (basic one-step *kumite*) is a training method designed to help practitioners master a range of basic technical skills, such as body shifting, proper stances, and offensive and defensive technical abilities.

When practicing *kihon ippon-kumite* special care needs to be taken to ensure that movements are performed correctly, with proper breathing and posture, otherwise technique, power, and spirit will be sacrificed. Maintaining proper posture not only relaxes the body, it conveys refinement, dignity, formality, and aesthetic appeal.

For more advanced practitioners this training method is also well suited to the development of *zanshin* (a state of physical and mental preparedness), *sahō* (etiquette), and the ability to "read" an opponent's breathing and movement.

In *kihon ippon-kumite* the attacking technique and target are predetermined and attacks are launched one at a time. Upon facing one another both participants stand up straight in *musubi-dachi* (closed V stance), bow once, and then shift into *hachiji-dachi shizentai* (open V stance) while looking into each other's eyes. The attacker then draws the right (or left) foot back one step into *zenkutsu-dachi* (front stance) while executing a left (or right) *gedan-barai* (downward block). The attacker, after informing the defender of the target, then concentrates the focus in his lower abdomen and launches a forceful attack with the intent of felling his opponent with a single strike.

When attacking, of greater importance than the posture while in the ready position is the ability to read an opponent's breathing, locate an opportunity to attack, and then swiftly take advantage of it.

The defender must maintain a level of spirit that exceeds that of the attacker, exercising patience while awaiting the attacker's strike. As the attack begins the defender must simultaneously move in the proper direction while effectively blocking and assuming a proper stance, and then promptly deliver a counterattack.

Following the defender's counterattack the attacker quietly returns to *hachiji-dachi shizentai* while breathing in, then exhales deeply while concentrating the focus in his lower abdomen, and relaxes in preparation for the next attack.

As in *gohon kumite* (five-step *kumite*) and *sanbon kumite* (three-step *kumite*), after delivering the final punch or strike of the counterattack, the defender maintains the completed position for two to three seconds. This serves to train and develop the muscles used when performing the technique. The recovery following the counterattack also provides an opportunity for the defender to further develop *zanshin*, *sahō*, and the ability to read an opponent's breathing and movement. As the attacker quietly returns to *hachiji-dachi shizentai*, the defender moves in synchronization, inhaling while returning to *hachiji-dachi shizentai*, and then exhaling while tightening his body. During this motion, it is important to remain as relaxed as possible. The defender must strive to achieve harmony with the attacker in terms of movement, breathing, and use of strength, constantly looking deep into the attacker's eyes while doing so.

The repeated practice of *kihon ippon-kumite* enables the mastery of not only *zanshin* and *sahō*, it also supports the future development of the ability to "read" an opponent's moves.

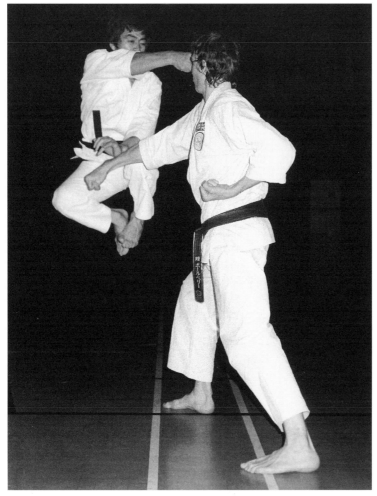

Delivering a jumping punch.

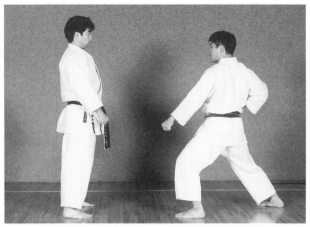
1

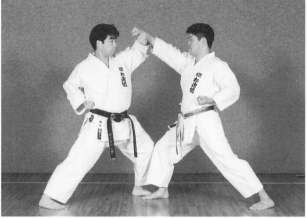
2

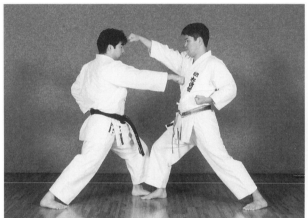
3

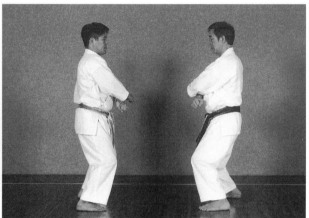
4

Jōdan Oi-Zuki (Upper-Level Lunge Punch) No. 1

1–2. When the attacker (right) begins from a *hidari gedan-barai* (left downward block) ready position (photo 1), the defender steps back with the right foot while simultaneously blocking with *age-uke* (rising block) (photo 2).

2. To ensure an effective block, sharply pull the right hip and right shoulder back when performing *age-uke* so that the hips and shoulders end up at a 45-degree angle to the front. The rotation of the hips and the twisting of the wrist of the blocking arm are executed simultaneously.

3. Utilizing the reaction from the block, the defender counters with *chūdan gyaku-zuki* (middle-level reverse punch).

4. Attacker and defender recover.

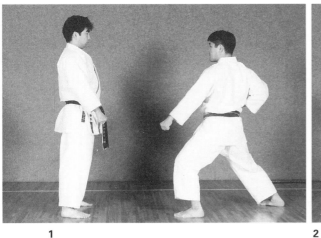

1

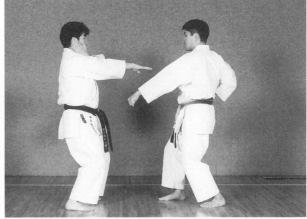

2

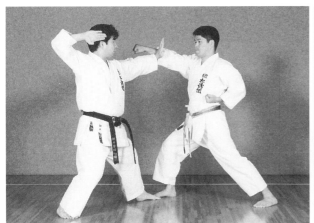

3

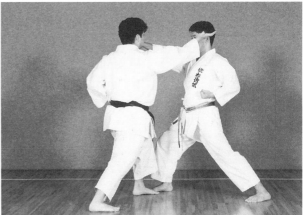

4

Jōdan Oi-Zuki No. 2

1–3. When the attacker (right) begins from a *hidari gedan-barai* ready position (photo 1), the defender steps back with the right foot at a 45-degree angle to the right into *kōkutsu-dachi* (back stance) while simultaneously blocking with *hidari jōdan tate shutō-uke* (upper-level vertical knife-hand block) (photos 2 and 3). The *hiki-te* (pulling hand; right hand in photo) is drawn back with the feeling of striking to the rear with the elbow.

4. The defender immediately thrusts off of the rear foot (right foot in photo) shifting into *zenkutsu-dachi* (front stance) while simultaneously countering with *jōdan shutō-uchi* (upper-level knife-hand strike).

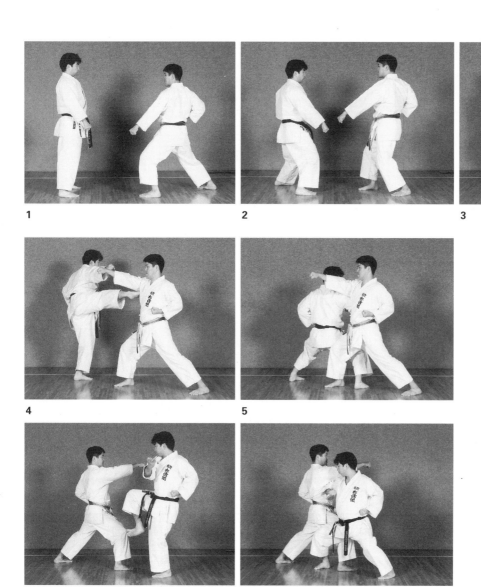

1

2

3

4

5

4′

5′

Jōdan Oi-Zuki No. 3

1–3. When the attacker (right) begins from a *hidari gedan-barai* ready position (photo 1), the defender slides his left foot outward diagonally to the left (photo 2). The right foot is immediately drawn in toward the left foot while simultaneously blocking with *sokumen jōdan uke* (side upper-level block) (photo 3).

4–5. The defender counters with *yoko-geri ke-age* (side snap kick), then steps inward with the kicking foot (right foot in photo) into *kiba-dachi* (straddle-leg stance), positioning his leg directly behind that of the attacker while simultaneously executing *yoko empi-uchi* (side elbow strike). When stepping in, the defender should carry out the motion with the feeling of using his thigh to strike the thigh of the attacker.

4′. Reverse-angle view of form between photos 4 and 5 (after *yoko-geri ke-age* and before *yoko empi-uchi*).

5′. Reverse-angle view of photo 5 (*kiba-dachi, yoko empi-uchi*).

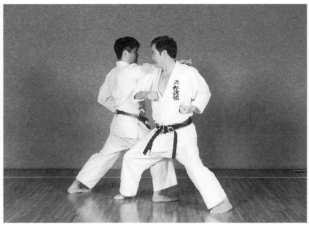

1

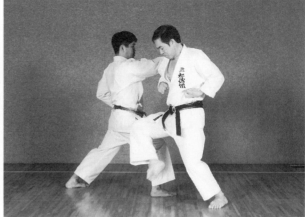

2

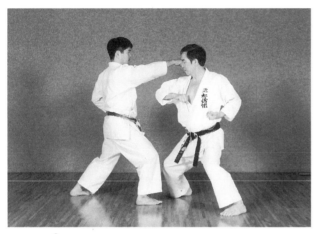

3

Jōdan Oi-Zuki No. 3—Supplement

1–2. Following the *yoko empi-uchi* counterattack by the defender (photo 1), both defender (right) and attacker step back, returning to their respective starting positions. When doing so, the defender withdraws the leg that is located behind the attacker (right leg in photo) with *nami-ashi* (inward foot snap) (photo 2) to ensure that it does not get snagged on the attacker's leg in the process.

3. Incorrect form. When stepping in following *yoko-geri ke-age* to execute *yoko empi-uchi*, the foot must be planted behind the attacker, as shown in photo 1.

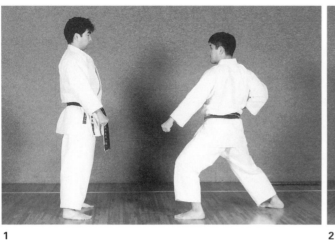

1

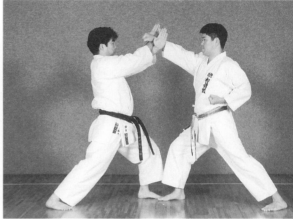

2

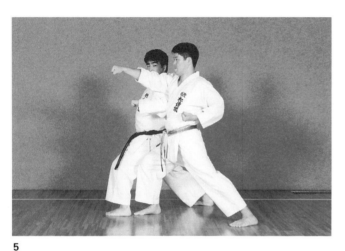

5

Jōdan Oi-Zuki No. 4

1–2. When the attacker (right) begins from a *hidari gedan-barai* ready position (photo 1), the defender steps back with the right leg while simultaneously blocking with *jōdan haishu juji-uke* (upper-level backhand X-block) (photo 2). When executing the block, the right hand is positioned in front of (above) the left hand.

3. The defender firmly grasps the attacker's wrist with his right hand and, keeping the elbow straight, extends his right arm out to the side while simultaneously countering with *mawashi-geri* (roundhouse kick). In doing so, the defender draws the attacker in by pulling the right hand toward the rear, utilizing the reaction to deliver the kick.

4–5. The defender retracts the kicking leg and places the foot on the outside of the attacker while rotating his body to the left and executing *hidari mawashi empi-uchi* (left roundhouse elbow strike).

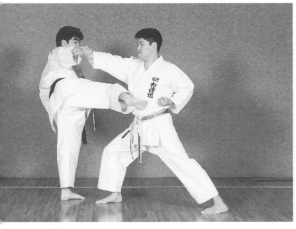

3

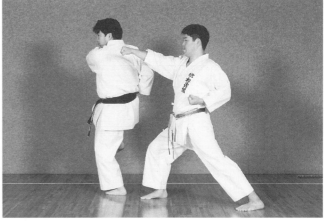

4

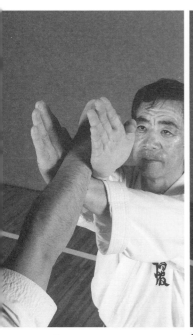

a

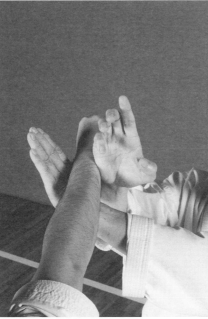

b

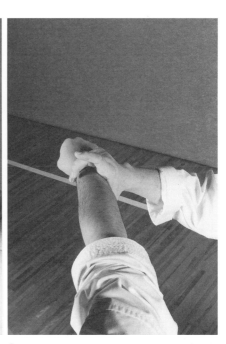

c

a. Close-up view of hand position for *jōdan haishu juji-uke*.

b. When turning the hand over to grasp the attacker's wrist, each finger is bent at a different angle as shown in photo 7. This enables the little finger to grab hold of the wrist first, followed by each of the other fingers in succession.

c. Close-up view of the right hand after it has taken hold of the attacker's wrist.

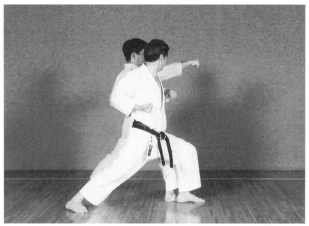

1

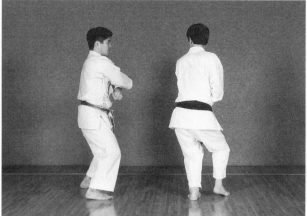

2

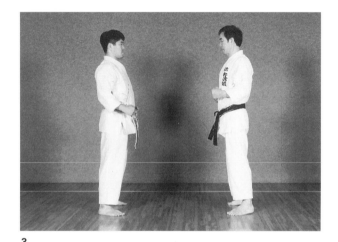

3

Jōdan Oi-Zuki No. 4—Supplement: Returning to the Starting Position

1. Step forward with the kicking leg, placing the foot on the outside of the attacker while rotating the body to the left and executing *hidari mawashi empi-uchi*.

2–3. Turn to the left (photo 2) and smoothly return to the starting position (photo 3).

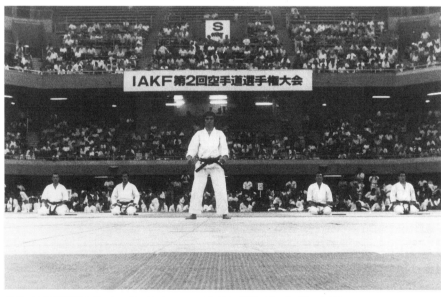

At the second IAKF karate championship tournament, held in 1977 at the Budōkan in Tokyo.

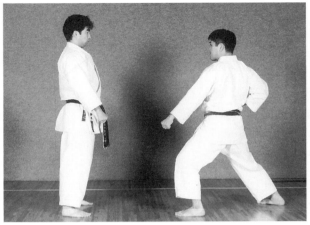

1

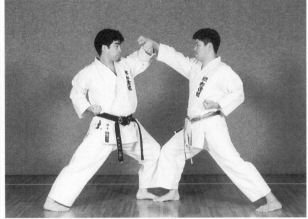

2

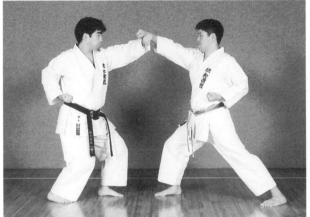

3

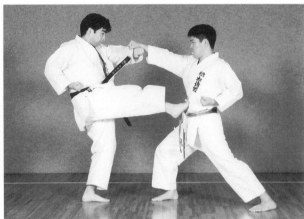

4

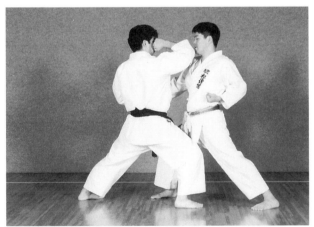

5

Jōdan Oi-Zuki No. 5

1–2. Kihon Ippon-Kumite/Jōdan Oi-zuki No. 5 begins in the same manner as No. 1, blocking with *jōdan age-uke*.

3. The defender draws his front foot (left foot in photo) back one-half step. When doing so, it is important that the hips remain at the same height.

4–5. The defender then counters with *migi mae-geri* (right front snap kick) (photo 4) and, stepping forward, follows through with *tate enmpi-uchi* (upward elbow strike) (photo 5).

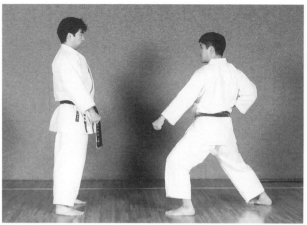

1

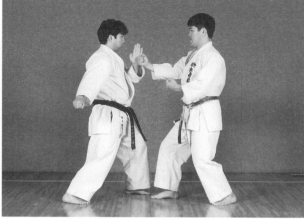

2

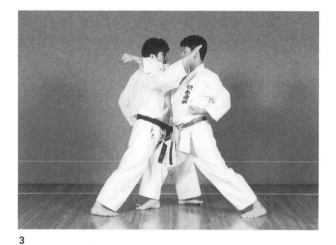

3

Jōdan Oi-Zuki No. 6

1–2. When the attacker (right) begins from a *hidari gedan-barai* ready position (photo 1), the defender steps back with the right foot while simultaneously blocking with *hidari hirate-barai* (left open-hand sweeping block) (photo 2).

3. Upon blocking, the left hand then becomes the *hiki-te*. Utilizing the reaction from the *hiki-te*, the defender rotates his hips while simultaneously executing *migi jōdan haitō-uchi* (right upper-level ridge-hand strike).

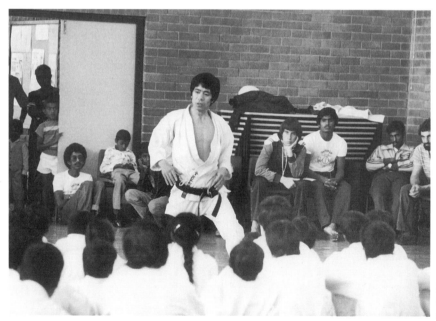

Explaining the proper use of the abdomen and knees in the United Arab Emirates.

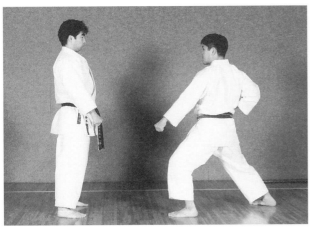

1

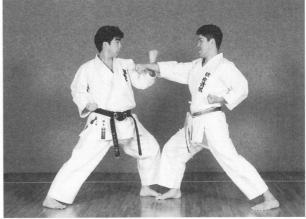

2

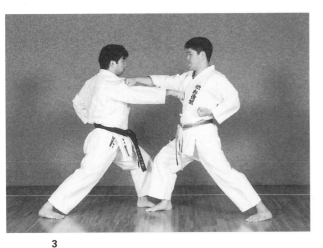

3

Chūdan Oi-Zuki (Middle-Level Lunge Punch) No. 1

1–2. When the attacker (right) begins from a *hidari gedan-barai* (left downward block) ready position (photo 1), the defender steps back with the right leg while simultaneously blocking with *hidari chūdan soto ude-uke* (left middle-level outside-to-inside block) (photo 2). To ensure an effective block, sharply pull the right hip and right shoulder back when performing *soto ude-uke*. The rotation of the hips and the twisting of the wrist of the blocking arm are executed simultaneously.

3. Utilizing the reaction from the block, the defender counters with *chūdan gyaku-zuki* (middle-level reverse punch).

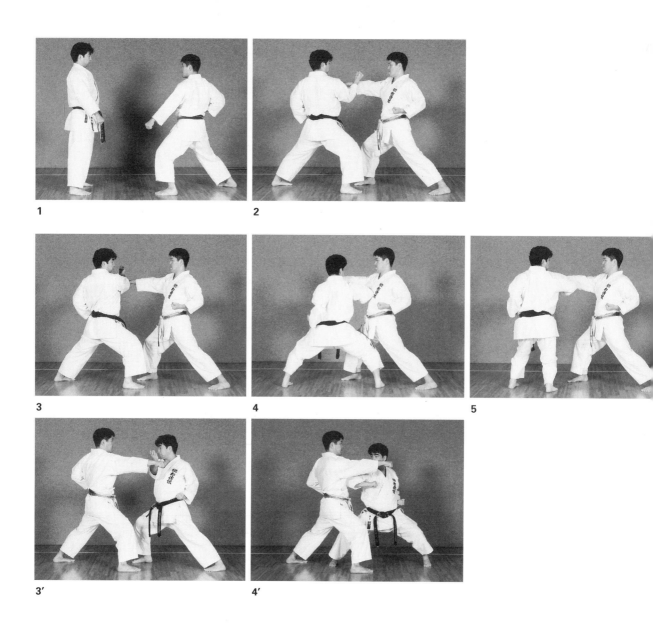

1   2

3   4   5

3'   4'

Chūdan Oi-Zuki No. 2

1–2. When the attacker (right) begins from a *hidari gedan-barai* ready position (photo 1), the defender, following the same principle as that for Kihon Ippon-Kumite/Chūdan Oi-zuki No. 1, steps back with the left foot while simultaneously blocking with *migi chūdan soto ude-uke* in *zenkutsu-dachi* (front stance) (photo 2).

3–4. The defender immediately moves forward with *suri-ashi* (a gliding step, without raising the foot), leading with the right foot, shifting into *kiba-dachi* (straddle-leg stance) while simultaneously countering with *yoko empi-uchi* (side elbow strike) (photo 4).

5. Following *kime* (execution of final technique with focus), the right foot is drawn back the distance that it slid forward during *suri-ashi* (photo 5), then the left foot is replaced to its original starting position and the defender returns to *shizentai* (natural posture).

3'. Reverse-angle view of photo 3.

4'. Reverse-angle view of photo 4 (*kiba-dachi, yoko empi-uchi*).

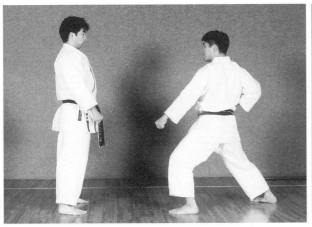

1

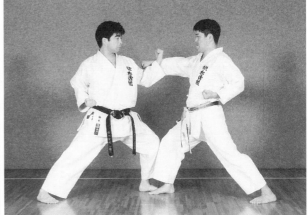

2

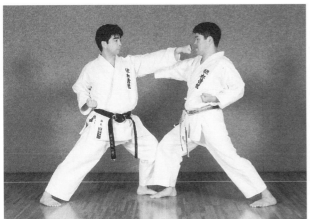

3

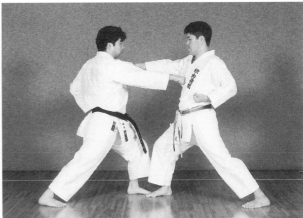

4

Chūdan Oi-Zuki No. 3

1–2. When the attacker begins from a *hidari gedan-barai* ready position (photo 1), the defender steps back with the right foot while simultaneously executing *chūdan uchi ude-uke* (middle-level inside-to-outside block) (photo 2). To ensure an effective block, sharply pull the right hip and right shoulder back when performing *uchi ude-uke*. The rotation of the hips and the twisting outward of the blocking arm are executed simultaneously.

3–4. The defender immediately counters with *jōdan kizami-zuki* (upper-level jab) (photo 3) followed by *chūdan gyaku-zuki* (photo 4).

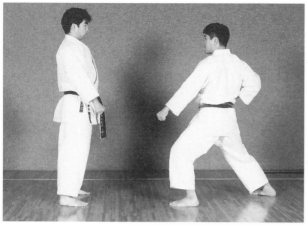

1

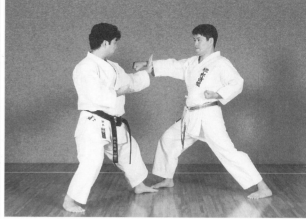

2

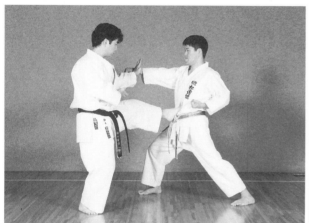

3-A

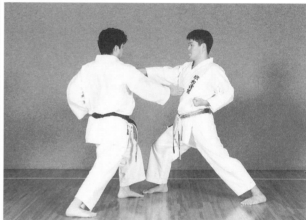

4

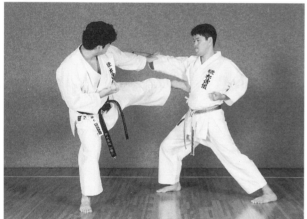

3-B

Chūdan Oi-Zuki No. 4

1–2. When the attacker (right) begins from a *hidari gedan-barai* ready position (photo 1), the defender steps back with the right foot at a 45-degree angle to the right into *kōkutsu-dachi* (back stance) while simultaneously blocking with *chūdan shutō-uke* (middle-level knife-hand block) (photo 2).

3-A. The defender counters with *chūdan kizami-geri* (middle-level short front kick).

3-B. Instead of *kizami-geri*, the defender may also use *kizami mawashi-geri* (short roundhouse kick). Which kick is selected will depend on the distance from the attacker following the block.

4. After the kick, the defender immediately thrusts off of the rear foot (right foot in photo) and shifts into *zenkutsu-dachi* while simultaneously following through with *chūdan tate shihon nukite* (middle-level vertical four-finger spear hand).

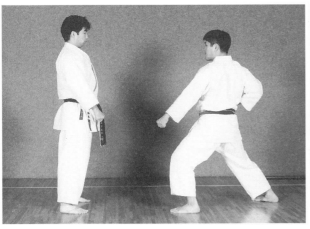

1

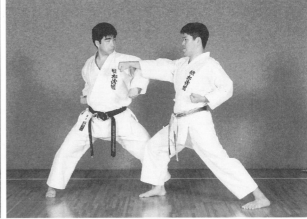

2

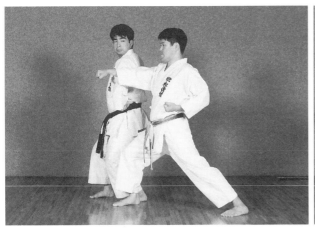

3

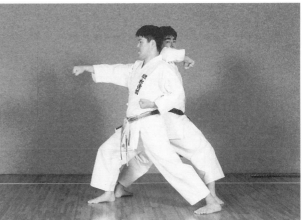

4

Chūdan Oi-Zuki No. 5

1–2. When the attacker (right) begins from a *hidari gedan-barai* ready position (photo 1), the defender steps back with the right leg into *kiba-dachi*, simultaneously blocking with *chūdan hiji-uke* (middle-level elbow block) (photo 2).

3–4. The defender, pivoting on the left foot (photo 3), turns 180 degrees clockwise (to the rear) into *kiba-dachi* while simultaneously countering with *jōdan ushiro mawashi empi-uchi* (upper-level back roundhouse elbow strike) (photo 4).

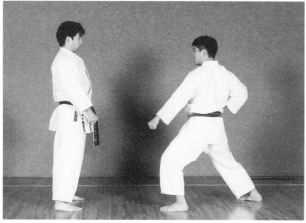

1

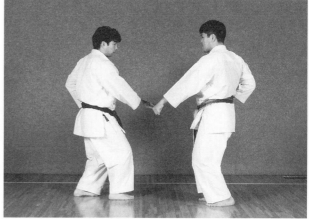

2

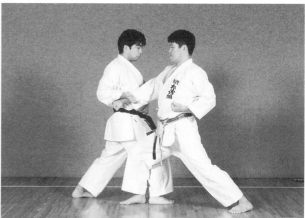

3

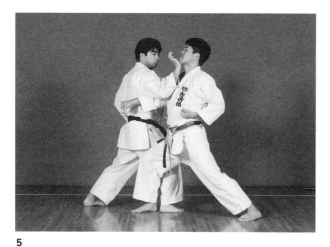

4

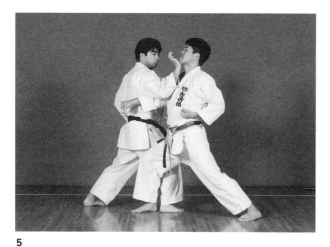

5

Chūdan Oi-Zuki No. 6

1–2. When the attacker (right) begins from a *hidari gedan-barai* ready position (photo 1), the defender steps forward with the right foot as the attacker moves forward to attack (photo 2).

3–4. Stepping so that the front foot passes along the outside of the attacker's front foot (photo 3), the defender blocks with *chūdan mawashi-uke* (middle-level round block) (photo 4).

5. The defender then counters with *jōdan tate teishō-uchi* (upper-level upward palm-heel strike).

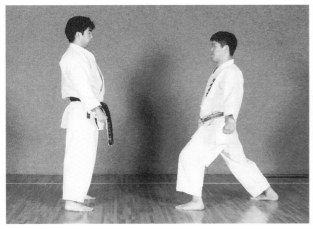

1

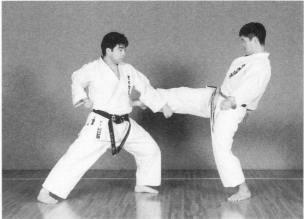

2

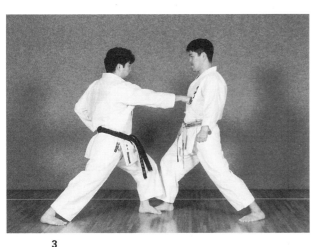

3

Mae-Geri (Front Snap Kick) No. 1

1–2. When the attacker (right) begins from a *hidari zenkutsu-dachi* (left front stance) ready position (photo 1), the defender steps back with the right leg while simultaneously blocking with *gedan-barai* (downward block) (photo 2). To ensure an effective block, sharply pull the right hip and right shoulder back when performing *gedan-barai*.

3. Utilizing the reaction from the block, the defender counters with *chūdan gyaku-zuki* (middle-level reverse punch).

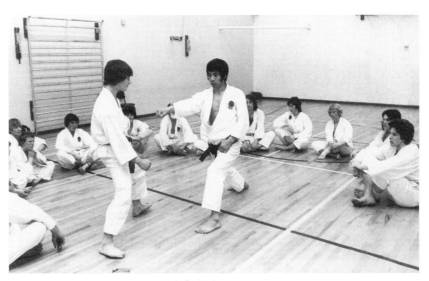

Explaining how to perform a reverse punch in England.

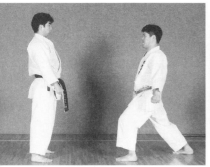

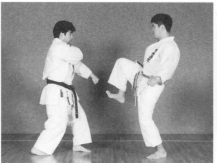

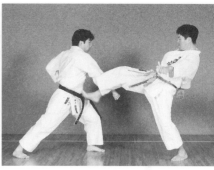

1 2 3

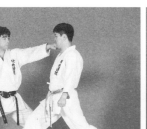

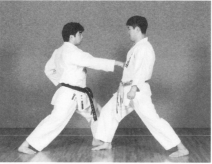

4 5

Mae-Geri No. 2

1–3. When the attacker (right) begins from a *hidari zenkutsu-dachi* ready position (photo 1), the defender steps back with the right foot while simultaneously blocking with *gyaku gedan-barai* (reverse downward block) (photo 3). To ensure an effective block, the blocking arm extends downward and to the front at a 45-degree angle.

4–5. The defender then immediately counters with *jōdan kizami-zuki* (upper-level jab) (photo 4) and follows through with *chūdan gyaku-zuki* (photo 5). When executing *kizami-zuki* and *gyaku-zuki*, it is important to utilize sufficient hip rotation.

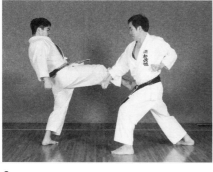

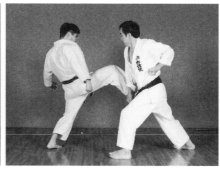

a b

Mae-Geri No. 2—Supplement: Gyaku Gedan-Barai

a. Correct form. The blocking arm extends downward at a 45-degree angle.

b. Incorrect form. The blocking arm extends straight down.

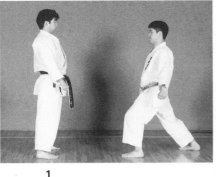 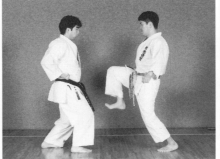 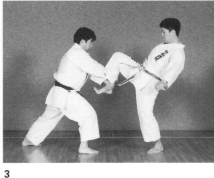

1 2 3

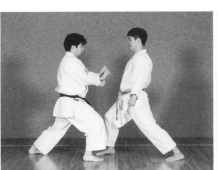 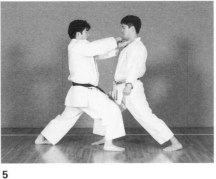 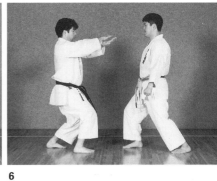

4 5 6

Mae-Geri No. 3

1–3. When the attacker (right) begins from a *hidari zenkutsu-dachi* ready position (photo 1), the defender steps back with the left foot (photo 2) while simultaneously blocking with *gedan jūji-uke* (lower-level X-block) (photo 3).

4–5. In preparation for the counterattack, the defender pulls in his elbows while keeping the fists crossed (photo 4), then immediately thrusts off the rear foot (left foot in photo) while executing *jōdan shutō jūji-uchi* (upper-level knife-hand X-strike) (photo 5). Special attention must be paid to the rotation of the arms when performing this technique.

6. The defender takes an extended breath (breathing in) while returning to the original starting position.

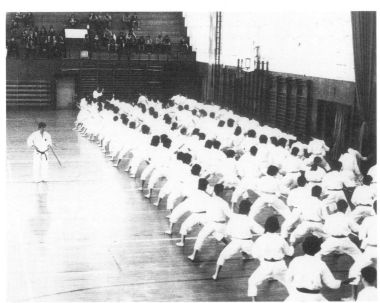

The author leading a training session in France.

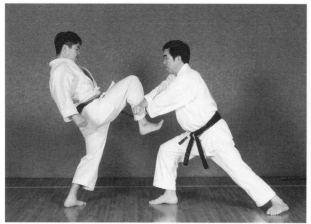

1

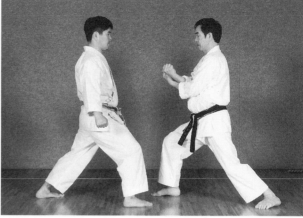

2

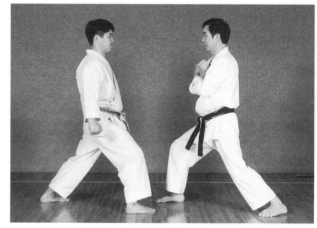

2'

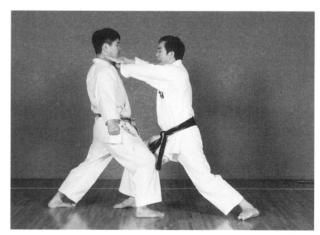

3

Mae-Geri No. 3—Supplement

1. *Gedan jūji-uke.*

2. Correct form. Prior to the counterattack, the defender's fists are aimed at the intended target.

2'. Incorrect form. The fists are pulled back to the chest and not pointing toward the target.

3. *Jōdan shutō jūji-uchi.*

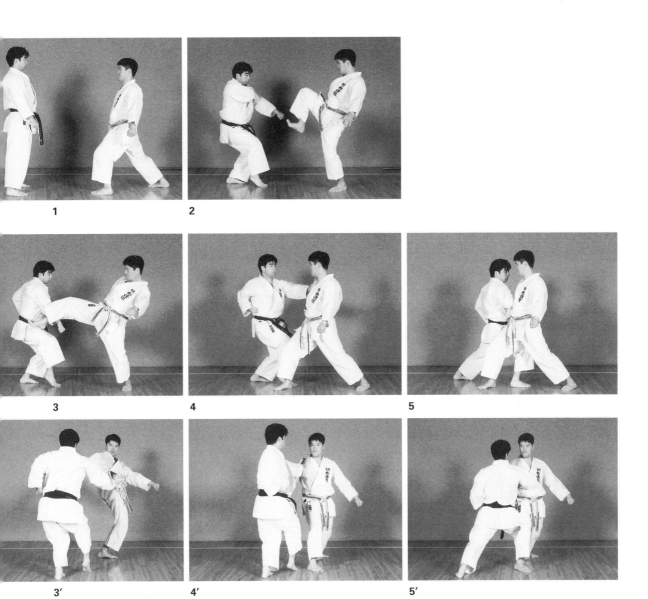

1   2

3   4   5

3'   4'   5'

Mae-Geri No. 4

1–3. When the attacker (right) begins from a *hidari zenkutsu-dachi* ready position (photo 1), the defender draws the right foot inward into *neko ashi-dachi* (cat stance) (photo 2) while simultaneously blocking with *migi gedan-barai* (photo 3).

4–5. The defender immediately steps forward with the right foot into *zenkutsu-dachi* while simultaneously countering with *mae empi-uchi* (forward elbow strike) (photo 5). In preparation for the counterattack, the *uke-te* (blocking hand; right hand in photo) is drawn back while the left hand is thrust out toward the attacker in tate *shutō* (vertical knife-hand) (photo 4).

3'–5'. Side-angle views of photos 3–5.

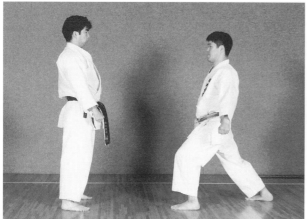

1

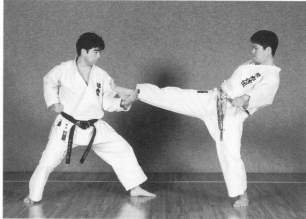

2

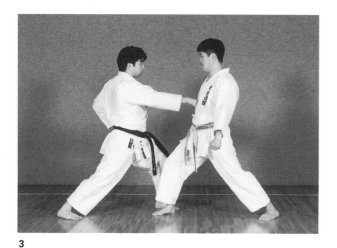

3

Mae-Geri No. 5

1–2. When the attacker (right) begins from a *hidari zenkutsu-dachi* ready position (photo 1), the defender steps back with the right leg into *kōkutsu-dachi*, catching the attacker's foot and drawing him in with *sukui-uke* (scooping block) (photo 2).

3. The defender immediately shifts into *zenkutsu-dachi* while simultaneously countering with *chūdan gyaku-zuki*.

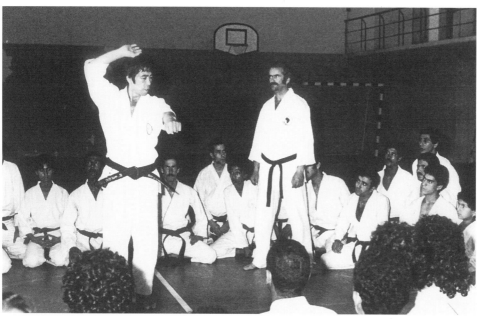

Explaining a blocking technique at a training session in Lebanon.

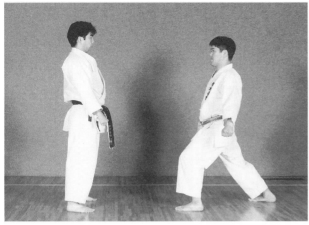

1

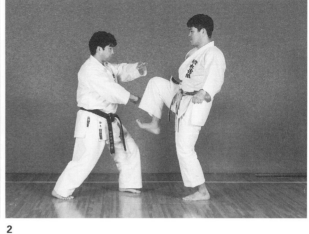

2

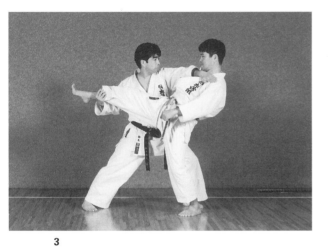

3

Mae-Geri No. 6

1–2. When the attacker (right) begins from a *hidari zenkutsu-dachi* ready position (photo 1), the defender steps forward with the left foot while blocking with *gyaku gedan-uke* (reverse downward block) using the right arm (photo 2).

3. With the left hand positioned at the attacker's neck and the right hand hooked under the kicking leg (photo 3), the defender throws the attacker over.

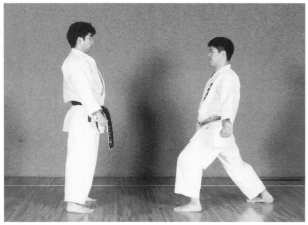

1

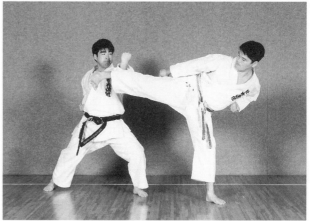

2

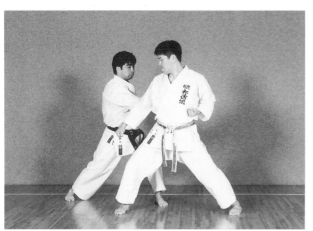

3

Yoko-Kekomi (Side Thrust Kick) No. 1

1–2. When the attacker (right) begins from a *hidari zenkutsu-dachi* (left front stance) ready position (photo 1), the defender, pivoting on the left foot, steps back and to the left with the right foot at a 45-degree angle, sharply rotating the hips while blocking with *chūdan soto ude-uke* (middle-level outside-to-inside block) (photo 2).

3. The defender immediately counters with *chūdan gyaku-zuki* (middle-level reverse punch).

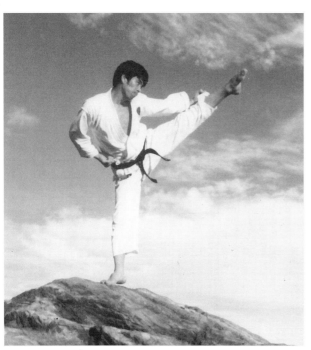

The author demonstrates a side kick on a cliff in Hawaii.

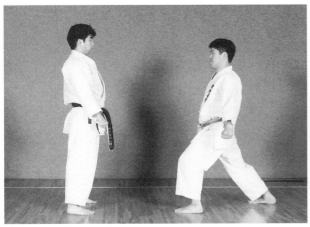

1

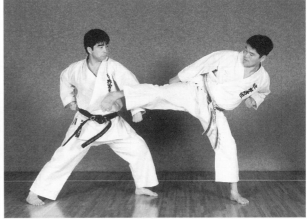

2

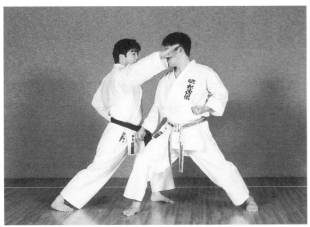

3

Yoko-Kekomi No. 2

1–2. When the attacker (right) begins from a *hidari zenkutsu-dachi* ready position (photo 1), the defender steps back with the right foot into *fudō-dachi* (rooted stance) while blocking with *chūdan haiwan-uke* (middle-level back-arm block) (photo 2).

3. The defender immediately counters with *jōdan haitō-uchi* (upper-level ridge-hand strike) in *zenkutsu-dachi*, utilizing the twisting of the hips to generate momentum for an effective strike.

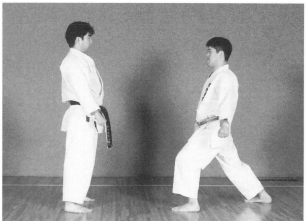

1

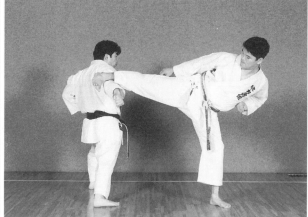

2

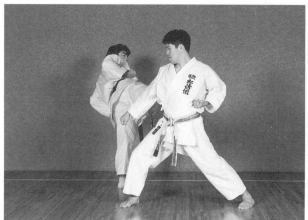

3

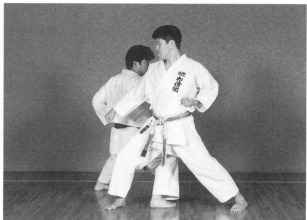

4

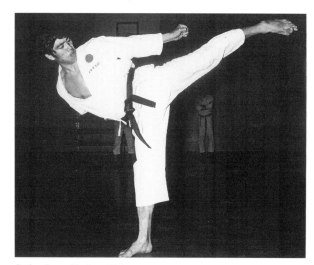

Performing a side thrust kick.

Yoko-Kekomi No. 3

1–2. When the attacker (right) begins from a *hidari zenkutsu-dachi* ready position (photo 1), the defender steps out to the left side with the left foot into *zenkutsu-dachi* (front stance) while blocking with *ushiro chūdan-barai* (back middle-level block) (photo 2).

3. From *zenkutsu-dachi*, the defender immediately counters with *chūdan yoko-kekomi* (middle-level side thrust kick).

4. The defender then follows through with *chūdan yoko empi-uchi* (middle-level side elbow strike) in *kiba-dachi* (straddle-leg stance).

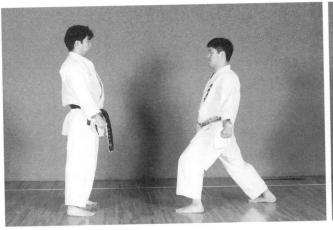

1

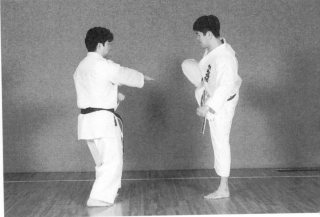

2

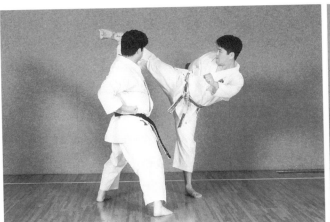

3

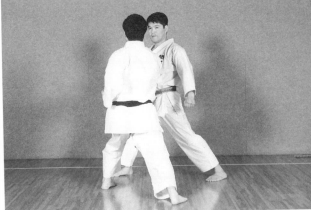

4

Mawashi-Geri (Roundhouse Kick) No. 1

1–3. When the attacker (right) begins from a *hidari zenkutsu-dachi* (left front stance) ready position (photo 1), the defender steps out to the right with the right foot into *zenkutsu-dachi* while blocking with *jōdan haiwan-uke* (upper-level back-arm block) (photo 3).

4. The defender immediately counters with *chūdan gyaku-zuki* (middle-level reverse punch).

4′. Side-angle view of photo 4.

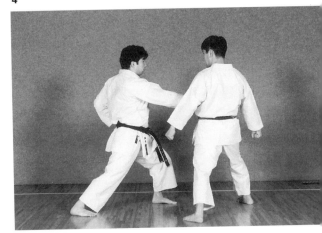

4′

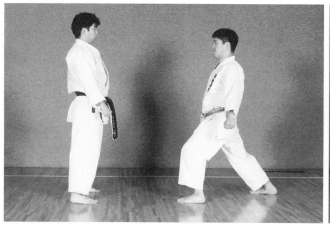

1

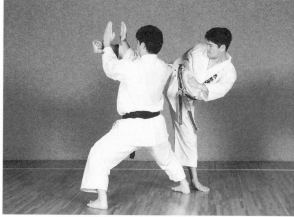

2

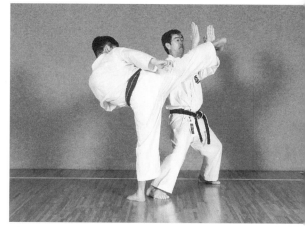

2'

Mawashi-Geri No. 2

1–2. When the attacker (right) begins from a *hidari zenkutsu-dachi* ready position (photo 1), the defender, pivoting on the right foot, revolves 135 degrees counterclockwise (to the rear) into *kiba-dachi* (back stance) while blocking with *tate heikō shutō-uke* (vertical parallel knife-hand block) (photo 2).

3. The defender immediately counters with *yoko empi-uchi* (side elbow strike), shifting in toward the attacker with *suri-ashi* (gliding step), leading with the right foot. When striking with *yoko empi-uchi*, the back of the right fist faces upward and the left hand is open, with the palm pressed against the front of the right fist to provide support.

2'–3'. Reverse-angle views of photos 2 and 3.

4'–6'. After the counterattack, the defender draws back the right foot one-half step (photo 4) and then, pivoting on the right foot, revolves 135 degrees clockwise (to the front) (photo 5), replacing the left foot to its original starting position (photo 6').

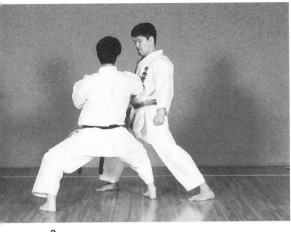

3

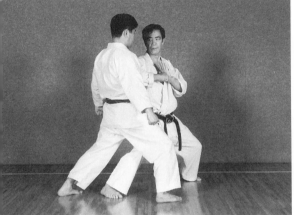

3′

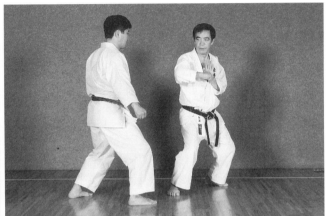

4′

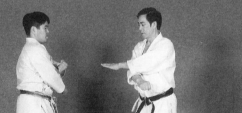

5′

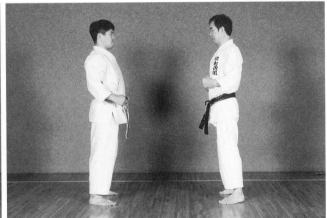

6′

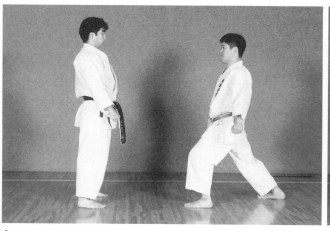

1

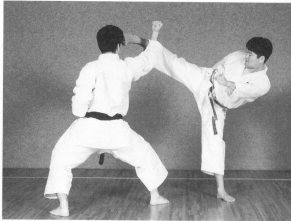

2

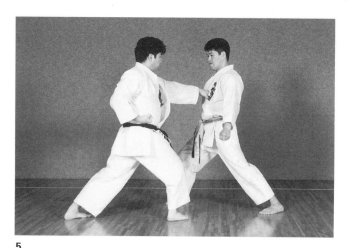

5

Mawashi-Geri No. 3

1–2. When the attacker (right) begins from a *hidari zenkutsu-dachi* ready position (photo 1), the defender, pivoting on the right foot, revolves 135 degrees counterclockwise (to the rear) into *kōkutsu-dachi* while blocking with *jōdan soto ude-uke* (upper-level outside-to-inside block) (photo 2).

3–5. The defender immediately counters with *chūdan kizami-geri* (middle-level short front kick) (photo 3) and follows through with *chūdan gyaku-zuki* in *zenkutsu-dachi* (photo 5).

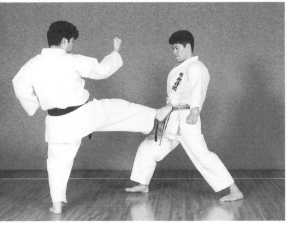

3

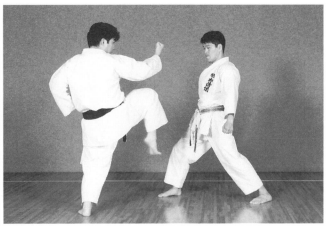

4

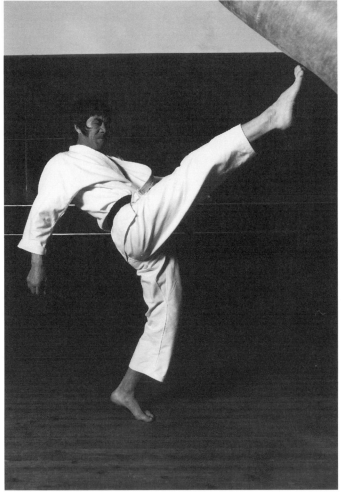

Performing a front snap kick.

KAESHI IPPON-KUMITE (Attack & Counter One-Step Kumite)

Kaeshi ippon-kumite (attack & counter one-step *kumite*) shares a sibling relationship with *kihon ippon-kumite* (basic one-step *kumite*). The objectives of both are basically the same. *Kaeshi ippon-kumite* combines the technical abilities developed through *tanren kumite* (training *kumite*) and the patterns of movement acquired through *kihon ippon-kumite* (basic one-step *kumite*) with the "feel" that comes through training in both types of *kumite*. As in *kihon ippon-kumite*, the defender must carefully observe his opponent and react accordingly the very instant that his opponent begins to move, properly blocking the attack and then instantly stepping forward while launching a counterattack at will. The attacker steps back or to the side and blocks the defender's counterattack, following through with a counterattack as in *jiyū ippon-kumite* (free-style one-step *kumite*).

One major characteristic that distinguishes *kaeshi ippon-kumite* from other types of *kumite* is that the initial attacker delivers the final counterattack. Additionally, with *gohon kumite* (five-step *kumite*), *sanbon kumite* (three-step *kumite*) and *kihon ippon-kumite*, after both attacker and defender initially face each other standing in *shizentai* (natural posture), the attacker draws one foot back into *zenkutsu-dachi* (front stance) while executing *gedan-barai* (downward block), the ready position from which the attack begins. With *kaeshi ippon-kumite*, however, the attacker launches his attack directly from the *shizentai* position.

One of the most important factors in martial arts is leg movement. Training in *kaeshi ippon-kumite* is well suited for developing the leg strength, agility, and quickness of movement necessary for the mastery of effective leg movement. Older karate practitioners, however, should exercise caution as this training is quite strenuous.

Physical readiness (*mi-gamae*), which concurs with maintaining proper health, represents the foundation on which all karate techniques are based and also facilitates a relaxed state of mind.

When performing *kaeshi ippon-kumite*, both practitioners stand in *shizentai* in *hachiji-dachi* (open V stance), applying their weight on the big toes and the inside edges of the feet in a relaxed posture. Each keeps his back straight and extended, and concentrates the focus in the lower abdomen.

The initial attacker informs his opponent of the intended target, and then, from the *shizentai* position, steps forward while delivering an attack. If, for example, the initial attacker announces *jōdan* (upper level) or *chūdan* (middle level) as his target, he would be free to use either his left or right fist, or *gyaku-zuki* (reverse punch), as long as the strike was aimed at the location that was stated. If, however, the attacker intends to use a kicking technique, he must inform his opponent of the type of kick that will be used.

The initial attacker must deliver his strike properly and forcefully. Just as in *kihon ippon-kumite*, the defender must effectively block the attack while assuming a proper stance, and then launch a counterattack. Unlike other types of *kumite*, however, in which the counterattack is executed from the position where the block was performed, the defender delivers the counterattack moving one step forward.

The initial attacker must move either straight back or to one side while simultaneously blocking his opponent's counterattack, and then deliver a counterattack of his own. Immediately after decisively executing the final counterattack, the initial attacker assumes a free-sparring stance, as is also the case following the counterattack when practicing *jiyū ippon-kumite*.

When performing *kaeshi ippon-kumite*, both attacker and defender must maintain a high level of spirit throughout their bodies. Each must carefully and patiently observe his opponent and be ready to promptly react at the first sign of movement, establishing proper *maai* (the distance maintained between opponents during *kumite*) while moving and firmly blocking each oncoming attack, and then following through with a counterattack.

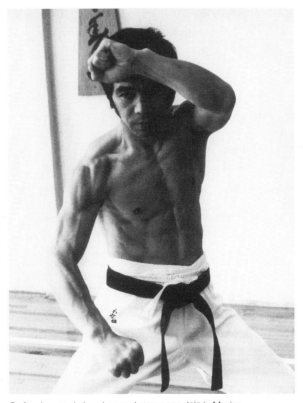

Performing a technique in rooted stance at a dōjō in Mexico.

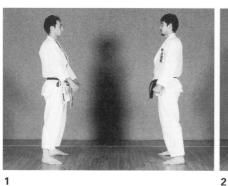

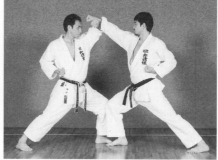

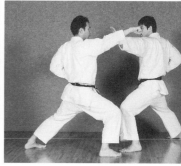

1   **2**   **3**

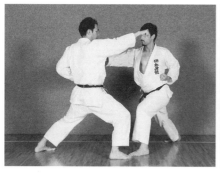

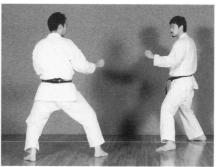

4   **5**

Kaeshi Ippon-Kumite A

In *kaeshi ippon-kumite,* the initial attacker (opponent B in photos) becomes the defender and executes the final counterattack in each exchange. The aim of this type of *kumite* is to develop agility and quickness when initiating a technique.

1. Opponent A (left) and opponent B face off in *shizentai* (natural posture).
2. A steps back, blocking with *jōdan age-uke* (upper-level rising block). / B steps forward, attacking with *jōdan oi-zuki* (upper-level lunge punch).
3. A steps forward, countering with *jōdan oi-zuki.* / B steps back at a 45-degree angle, blocking with *tate shutō-uke* (vertical knife-hand block).
4. B counters with *chūdan gyaku-zuki* (middle-level reverse punch).
5. A and B recover; B maintains *zanshin* (a state of physical and mental preparedness following an attack).

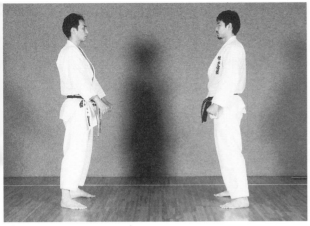

1

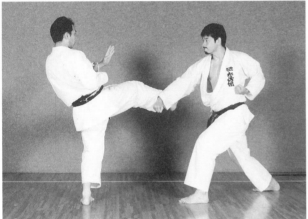

2

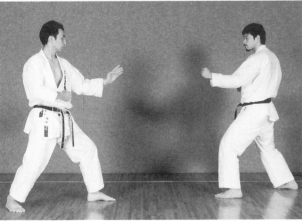

3

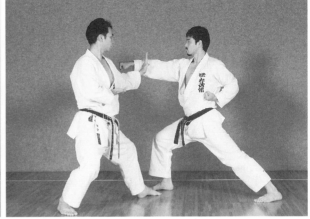

4

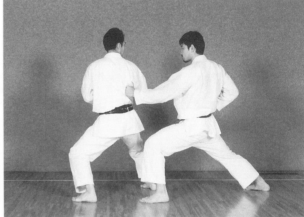

5

Kaeshi Ippon-Kumite B

1. Opponent A (left) and opponent B face off in *shizentai*.

2. A steps back at a 45-degree angle into *kōkutsu-dachi* (back stance), blocking with *shtō-uke*. / B steps forward, attacking with *chūdan oi-zuki*.

3. A steps forward, countering with *mae-geri* (front snap kick). / B steps back, blocking with *gyaku gedan-barai* (reverse downward block).

4. B counters with *chūdan kizami-zuki* (middle-level jab).

5. A and B recover; B maintains *zanshin*.

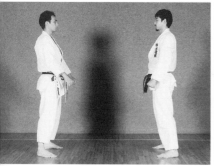

1

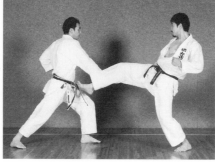

2

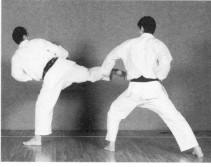

3

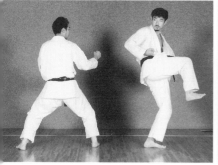

4

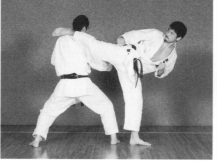

5

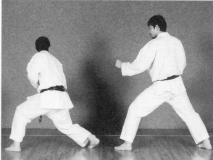

6

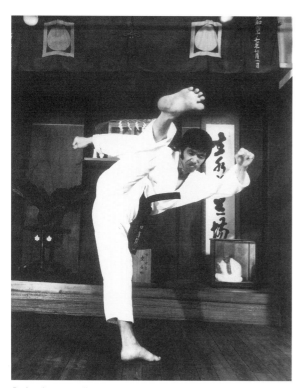

Performing a roundhouse kick at the Hōitsugan Dōjō.

Kaeshi Ippon-Kumite C

1. Opponent A (left) and opponent B face off in *shizentai*.

2. A steps back, blocking with *gyaku gedan-barai*. / B steps forward, attacking with *mae-geri*.

3. A steps forward, countering with *yoko-geri* (side kick). / B steps back, blocking with *haiwan-uke* (back-arm block).

4–5. Pivoting on the left foot (photo 4), B counters with *ushiro mawashi-geri* (back roundhouse kick) (photo 5).

6. A and B recover; B maintains *zanshin*.

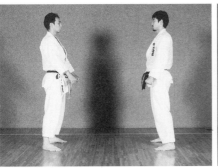

1

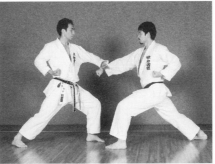

2

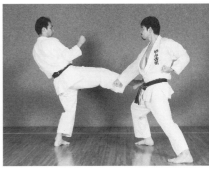

3

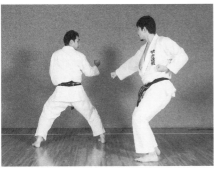

4

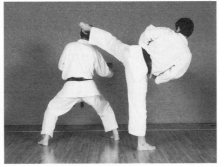

5

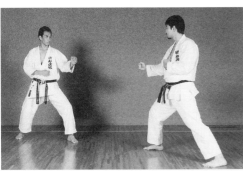

6

Kaeshi Ippon-Kumite D

1. Opponent A (left) and opponent B face off in *shizentai*.

2. A steps back, blocking with *gedan-barai* (downward block). / B steps forward, attacking with *chūdan gyaku-zuki*.

3. A steps forward, countering with *mae-geri*. / B steps back at a 45-degree angle, blocking with *gedan-barai*.

4–5. B draws the front foot back (photo 4) and counters with *jōdan mawashi-geri* (upper-level roundhouse kick) (photo 5).

6. A and B recover; B maintains *zanshin*.

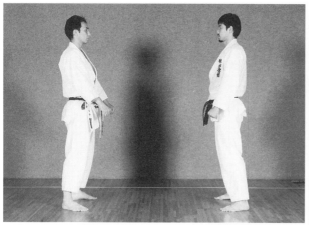

1

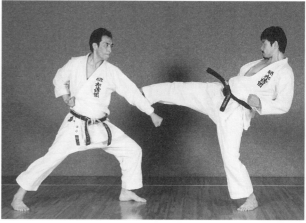

2

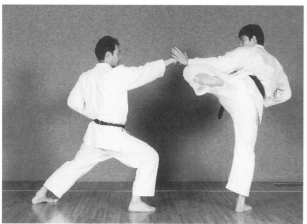

3

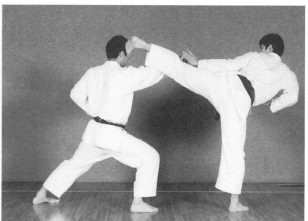

4

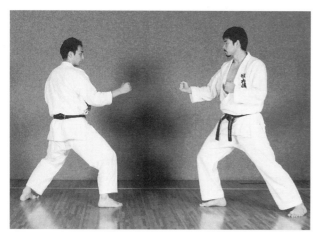

5

Kaeshi Ippon-Kumite E

1. Opponent A (left) and opponent B face off in *shizentai*.

2. A steps back, blocking with *gedan-barai*. / B steps forward, attacking with *mae-geri*.

3. A steps forward, countering with *jōdan oi-zuki*. / B steps back, blocking with *nagashi-uke* (sweeping block) while simultaneously lifting the front leg in preparation for a *mawashi-geri* counterattack.

4. B counters with *jōdan mawashi-geri*.

5. A and B recover; B maintains *zanshin*.

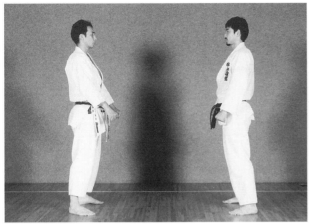

1

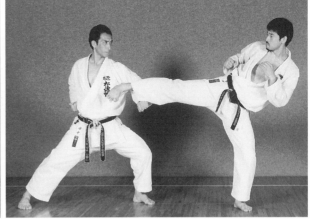

2

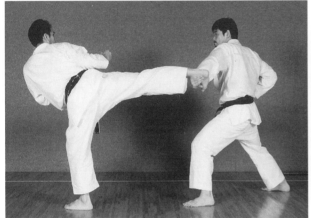

3

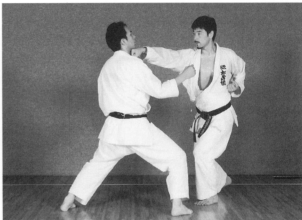

4

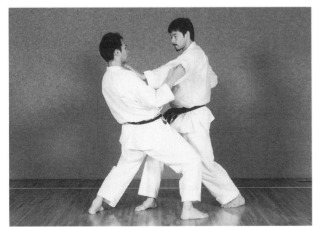

5

Kaeshi Ippon-Kumite F

1. Opponent A (left) and opponent B face off in *shizentai*.

2. A steps back, blocking with *haiwan-uke*. / B steps forward, attacking with *yoko-kekomi* (side thrust kick).

3. A steps forward, countering with *chūdan mawashi-geri*. / B steps back at a 45-degree angle blocking with *gedan-barai*.

4. B counters with *jōdan gyaku-zuki* while stepping forward.

5. B steps forward, using the left hand to keep A in check while maintaining *zanshin*.

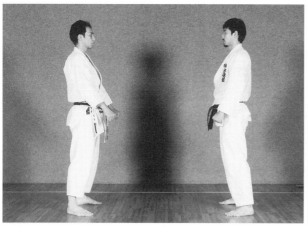

1

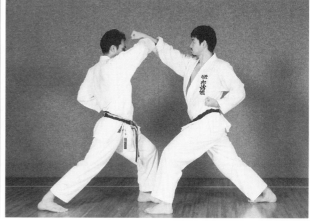

2

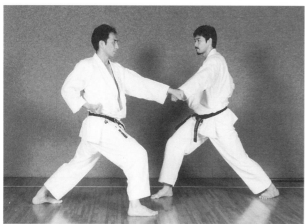

3

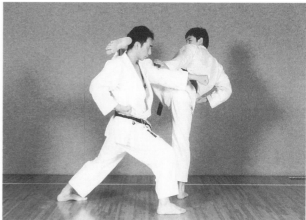

4

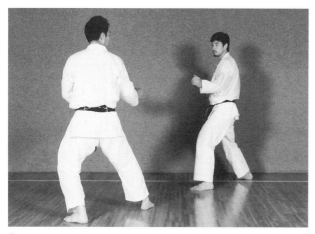

5

Kaeshi Ippon-Kumite G

1. Opponent A (left) and opponent B face off in *shizentai*.

2. A steps back, blocking with *gyaku age-uke* (reverse rising block). / B steps forward, attacking with *jōdan gyaku-zuki*.

3. A steps forward, countering with *chūdan gyaku-zuki*. / B steps back at a 45-degree angle blocking with *gyaku gedan-barai*.

4. B counters with *jōdan ushiro uchi mawashi-geri* (upper-level back inside roundhouse kick).

5. A and B recover; B maintains *zanshin*.

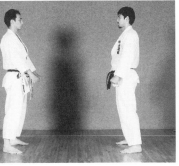 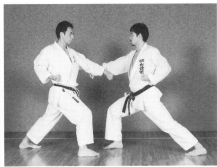 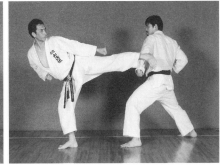

1   2   3

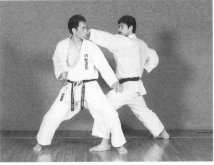 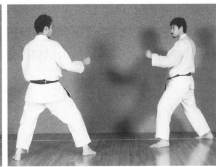

4   5   6

Kaeshi Ippon-Kumite H

1. Opponent A (left) and opponent B face off in *shizentai*.

2. A steps back, blocking with *gyaku gedan-barai*. / B steps forward, attacking with *chūdan oi-zuki*.

3. A steps forward, countering with *yoko-kekomi*. / B steps back at a 45-degree angle blocking with *gedan-barai*.

4–5. B draws the front foot back one-half step (photo 4) prior to lunging forward with *jōdan kizami-zuki* (photo 5).

6. A and B recover; B maintains *zanshin*.

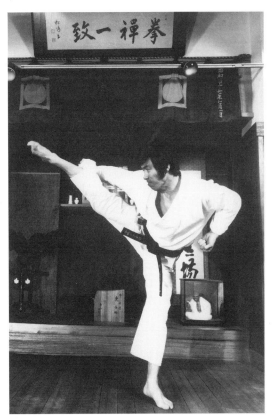

The author performs a side kick at the Hōitsugan Dōjō.

JIYŪ IPPON-KUMITE (Free-Style One-Step Kumite)

Jiyū ippon-kumite (free-style one-step *kumite*) represents a preparatory training for *jiyū kumite* (free-style *kumite*) that closely approximates the conditions of *jiyū-kumite*. Karate practitioners effectively apply the physical and mental strength, powerful stances, and fundamental technical abilities they have developed through *gohon kumite* (five-step *kumite*) and *sanbon kumite* (three-step *kumite*), along with the accurate offensive and defensive techniques and proper leg movements acquired through *kihon ippon-kumite* (basic one-step *kumite*) and *kaeshi ippon-kumite* (attack & counter one-step *kumite*). In *jiyū ippon-kumite*, the leg movement and body shifting that immediately follow the delivery of each counterattack are of particular importance.

Tanren kumite (training *kumite*) and *kihon kumite* (basic *kumite*) enable practitioners to develop the fundamental physical strength, posture, and range of correct technical capabilities essential for karate. But without the knowledge of how to use body shifting, body rotation, and *maai* (the distance maintained between opponents during *kumite*) in terms of both time and space, training in these types of *kumite* alone will not prove effective when facing a moving opponent.

As is evident when watching boxing, footwork and timing are extremely important. In the *kumite* of karate-dō, these factors take on even greater importance. Accordingly, special attention needs to be paid to thoroughly studying footwork and timing, and gaining practical experience through training.

In *tanren kumite* and *kihon kumite*, the defender uses his own strength to block his opponent's attack, and then launches a counterattack. In *jiyū ippon-kumite*, however, the defender takes advantage of his opponent's power, combining it harmoniously with his own strength and technical ability to shift his body in response to the attack, and then follow through with a counterattack. It is this aspect of *jiyū ippon-kumite* that distinguishes it from the training and basic types of *kumite*.

Expressed as a simple mathematical equation, the above concept would be written:

$$\text{Opponent's power} + \text{Own power} = \text{Harmonized power}$$

The sum of this formula translates into a counterattack of doubled strength. I believe this to be the true appeal of the *kumite* of karate-dō.

While *tanren kumite* and *kihon kumite* require that the *maai* remain constant, in *jiyū ippon-kumite*, the *maai* is more fluid and constantly changes during encounters.

The attacker informs his opponent of the target from a free-sparring stance and, when he feels that the *maai* and timing are appropriate, launches an attack. The defender shifts accordingly in response while blocking the attack, and then follows through with a counterattack. Or, the defender may simultaneously counter while shifting his body. Upon completing the counterattack the defender immediately distances himself from his opponent, or closes the distance by moving directly next to the attacker. If the defender remains in the same location from where he delivered the counterattack, he would be within easy striking range of the attacker. Ultimately, with each encounter, practitioners must determine how to make the most out of the single chance they have to either attack or defend.

The attacker must deliver his attack with the force and spirit intended by the expression "to kill with a single blow." The defender must carefully observe his opponent's movement, or must wait until the last possible moment before instantaneously shifting and countering.

When shifting the body, it is important to clearly distinguish between the pivoting foot and the foot that moves, maintaining the feeling that a single piece of paper is all that separates the bottom of the moving foot from the floor.

In *yakusoku kumite* (promise sparring), as in *tanren kumite* and *kihon kumite*, the attacker clearly states the target prior to launching his attack. Should the defender fail to block the attack, or block too late, and contact is made, the attacker would be free from any responsibility. If the defender, fully aware of the target and technique, were not to block correctly, only he would be at fault. It is only when this attitude is maintained by both practitioners during training that any significant improvement can be achieved. Of course exceptions must be made for differences in technical ability, age and strength.

When experienced practitioners engage in *jiyū ippon-kumite*, the attacker will read his opponent's breathing. For example, he may time his attack for the instant that the defender begins to inhale. He may also employ such techniques as feints and false starts to break his opponent's concentration or catch him off-balance.

Conversely, the defender must not allow his breathing to be read by the attacker. This can be achieved by maintaining proper posture and using the abdomen to control breathing. The defender must also not be fooled by such tricks as the use of feints by his opponent. This requires the development of a level of mental fortitude enabling him to wait until the last possible instant before the attacker's strike makes contact, and sufficient training in the use of body rotation and body shifting.

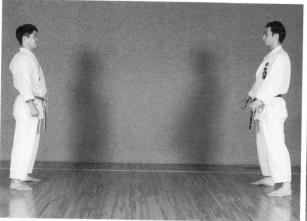

1

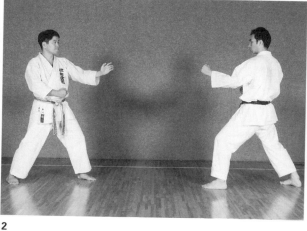

2

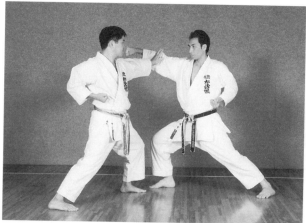

3

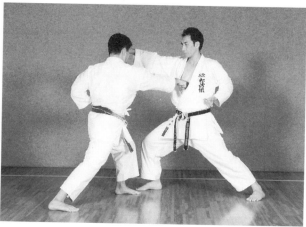

4

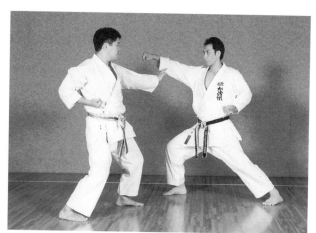

5

Jōdan Oi-Zuki
(Upper-Level Lunge Punch) No. 1

1–2. After the attacker (right) and defender have bowed to each other, they stand in *shizentai* (natural posture) (photo 1), and then assume a free-sparring stance (photo 2) when both are ready to commence.

3. Pivoting on the front foot (left foot in photo), the defender shifts 45 degrees to the right while blocking with *jōdan tate shutō-uke* (upper level vertical knife-hand block). The optimal location for the block is the crook of the attacker's arm.

4. Utilizing the reaction from the block, the defender immediately counters with *chūdan gyaku-zuki* (middle-level reverse punch).

5. When retracting the *tsuki-te* (punching hand; right hand in photo), the defender simultaneously draws the front foot (left foot in photo) back one-half step and assumes *hanmi* (half-front-facing position) *shizentai*.

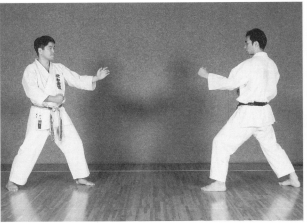

1

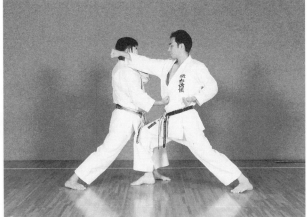

2

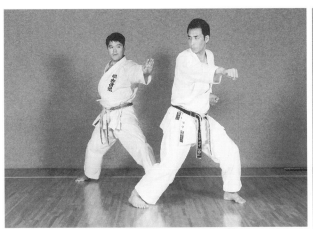

3

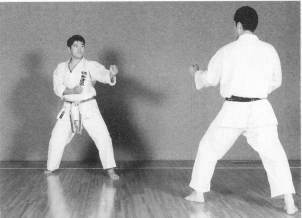

4

Jōdan Oi-Zuki No. 2

1. Attacker (right) and defender face off in free-sparring stance.

2. As the attacker commences his attack, the defender steps forward with the front foot (left foot in photo), blocking with *nagashi-uke* (sweeping block) while simultaneously countering with *chūdan gyaku ura-zuki* (middle-level reverse close punch). This counterattack is effective as it makes use of the "collision" resulting from the attacker and defender moving in from opposite directions.

3. The defender immediately pushes the attacker away using the blocking hand (left hand in photo) while shifting the back foot (right foot in photo) to the rear and left at a 45-degree angle.

4. Attacker and defender recover and assume free-sparring stances.

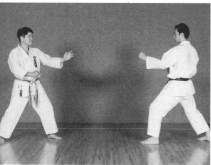
1

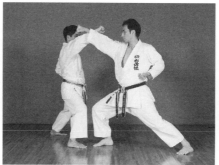
2

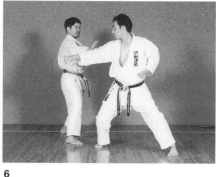
3

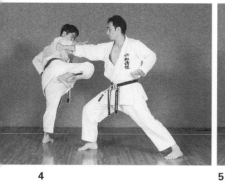
4

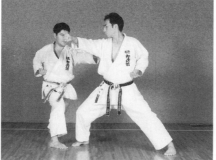
5

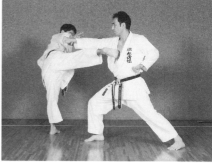
6

Jōdan Oi-Zuki No. 3

1. Attacker (right) and defender face off in free-sparring stance.

2. Pivoting on the back foot (right foot in photo), the defender retracts the front foot to the left and rear at a 45-degree angle while blocking with *jōdan age-uke* (upper-level rising block) in *zenkutsu-dachi* (front stance).

3–5. The defender immediately counters with *kizami mawashi-geri* (short roundhouse kick) (photo 3), followed by *chūdan gyaku-zuki* (photo 5).

6. When retracting the *tsuki-te* (left hand in photo), the defender simultaneously draws the front foot (right foot in photo) back one-half step and assumes *hanmi shizentai*.

Jōdan Oi-Zuki No. 4 (right page)

1. Attacker (right) and defender face off in free-sparring stance.

2. The defender steps to the outside with the front foot (left foot in photo) at a 45-degree angle while blocking with *jōdan hirate-barai* (upper-level open-hand sweeping block).

3. The defender counters with *chūdan teishō-uchi* (middle-level palm-heel strike).

4. After the counterattack, the defender, pivoting on the front foot (left foot in photo), shifts the back foot to the left while revolving 135 degrees clockwise.

5. Attacker and defender recover and assume free-sparring stances.

2'a. Side-angle view of photo 2.

2'b. Side-angle view showing hand position following block and prior to *chūdan teishō-uchi* counterattack.

3'–4'. Side-angle views of photos 3 and 4.

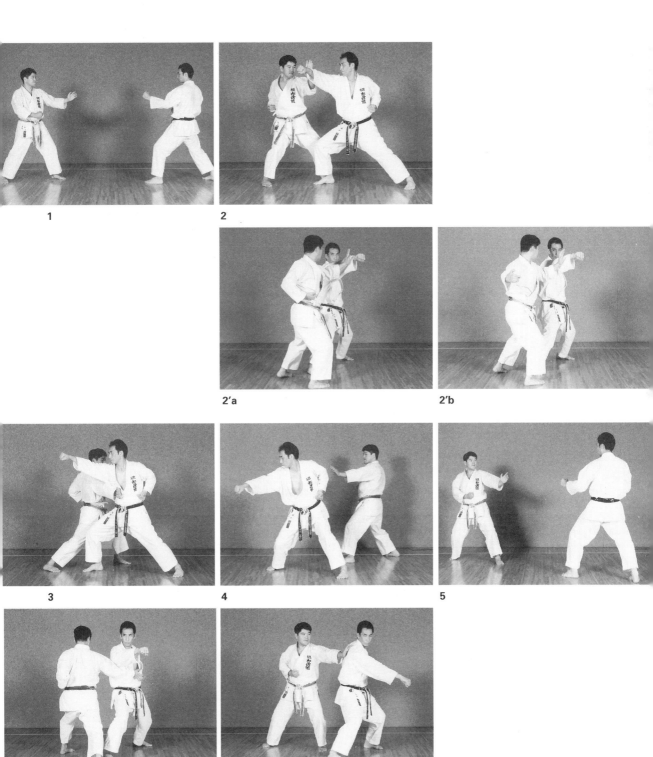

1

2

2'a

2'b

3

4

5

3'

4'

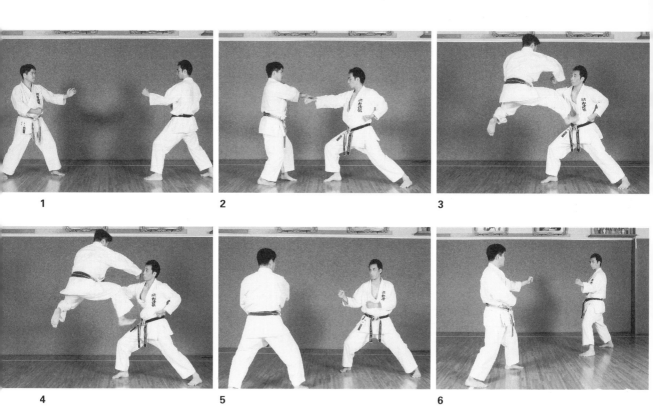

1 2 3

4 5 6

Jōdan Oi-Zuki No. 5

1. Attacker (right) and defender face off in free-sparring stance.

2. The defender draws the front foot (left foot in photo) back while blocking with *osae-uke* (pressing block).

3–4. The defender counters with *tobi-geri* (jump kick) (photo 3) and *jōdan yoko uraken-uchi* (upper-level side back-fist strike) (photo 4).

5–6. Upon landing (photo 5), the defender takes a step back and resumes a free-sparring stance (photo 6).

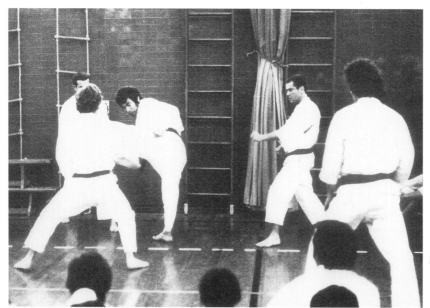

At a 1974 training session in Portugal.

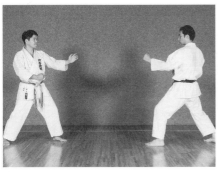

1

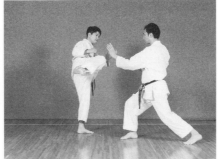

2

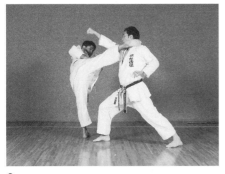

3

Jōdan Oi-Zuki No. 6

1. Attacker (right) and defender face off in free-sparring stance.

2–3. As the attacker approaches, the defender steps forward, shifting his body out of the path of the punch (photo 2), and counters with *jōdan mawashi-geri* (photo 3).

4–5. Following the kick, the defender steps forward (photo 4) and, pivoting on the front foot (right foot in photo), turns around to once again face the attacker in a free-sparring stance.

3'. The defender may also counter with *chūdan mawashi-geri*.

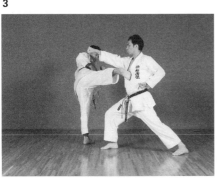

3'

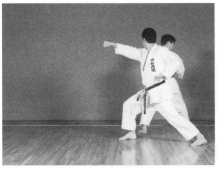

4

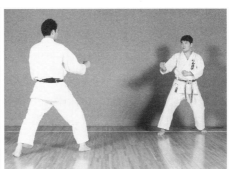

5

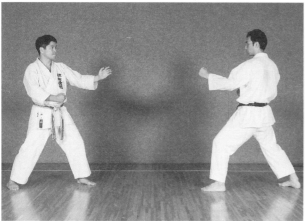

1

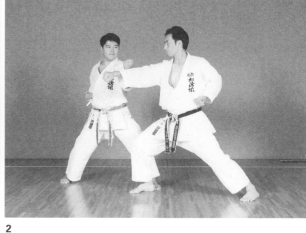

2

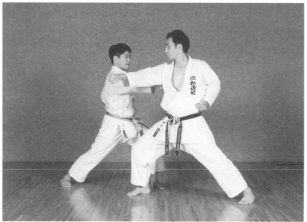

3

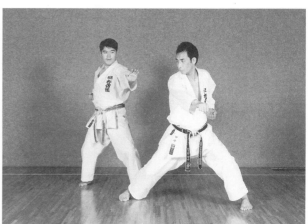

4

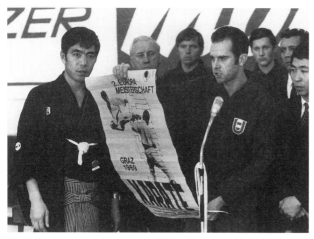

At the first European karate championship tournament, held in 1969 in Graz, Austria.

Chūdan Oi-Zuki
(Middle-Level Lunge Punch) No. 1

1. Attacker (right) and defender face off in free-sparring stance.

2. Pivoting on the front foot (left foot in photo), the defender shifts 45 degrees to the left while blocking with *chūdan soto ude-uke* (middle-level outside-to-inside block).

3. Utilizing the reaction from the block, the defender immediately counters with *chūdan gyaku-zuki* (middle-level reverse punch).

4. Following the counterattack, the defender, maintaining *zanshin* (a state of physical and mental preparedness following an attack), recovers by drawing the front foot back one-half step while deflecting the attacker's arm with the blocking hand.

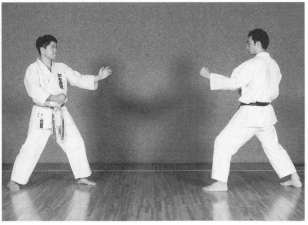

1

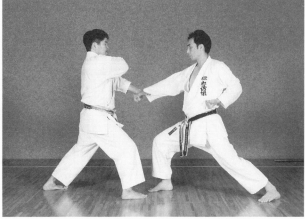

2

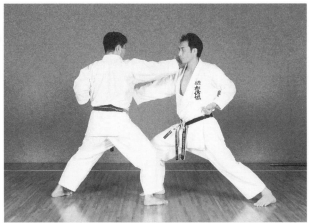

3

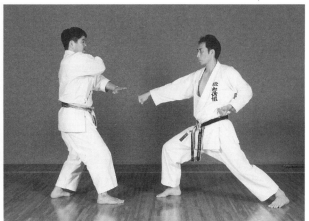

4

Chūdan Oi-Zuki No. 2

1. Attacker (right) and defender face off in free-sparring stance.

2. The defender, stepping straight back with the front foot (left foot in photo), blocks with *gedan seiryūtō-uke* (lower-level ox-jaw block). When blocking, the opposite hand forms a fist and is positioned above the left shoulder with the back of the hand facing outward.

3. The defender immediately counters with *jōdan uraken-uchi* (upper-level back-fist strike), thrusting off the back foot and utilizing hip rotation while simultaneously snapping from the elbow of the striking arm.

4. The defender, utilizing the reaction from the strike, shifts a half-step away from the attacker and draws the front foot back as he returns his hands and rotates the hips to the positions they were in prior to the counterattack.

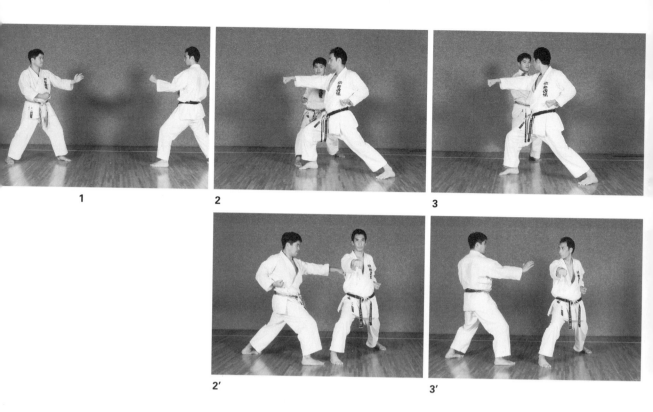

1 2 3

2' 3'

Chūdan Oi-Zuki No. 3

1. Attacker (right) and defender face off in free-sparring stance.
2. Pivoting on the back foot (right foot in photo), the defender draws the front foot directly out to the side, shifting out of the path of the attack without blocking while simultaneously executing *chūdan gyaku-zuki*.
3. The defender recovers and resumes a free-sparring stance, maintaining *zanshin*.

2'–3'. Rear-angle views of photo 2 and 3

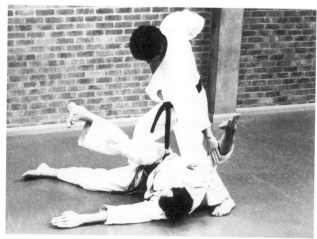

The author prepares to deliver a punch after throwing his opponent to the floor.

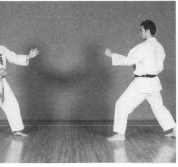 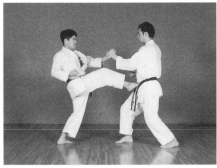 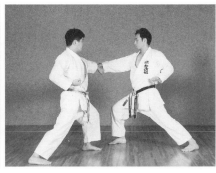

1   **2**   **3**

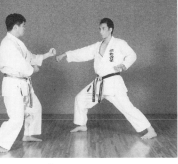 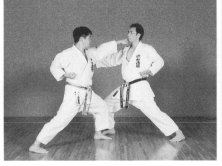 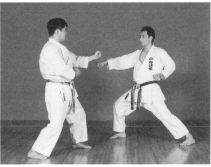

4   **5**   **6**

Chūdan Oi-Zuki No. 4

1. Attacker (right) and defender face off in free-sparring stance.

2. Before the attacker completes three-quarters of the step forward, the defender delivers *de-ai* (encounter) *chūdan mae-geri* (middle-level front snap kick) with the back leg (right leg in photo).

3. The defender pulls back the kicking leg, blocking with *gedan-barai* (downward block) as the pulling foot (*hiki-ashi*) is planted. Following the kick, the *hiki-ashi* is retracted to the right and rear so that the defender faces the attacker at an angle.

4–5. The defender draws the front foot back one-half step (photo 4) and immediately thrusts off the rear foot, countering with *jōdan kizami-zuki* (upper-level jab) (photo 5).

6. The defender recovers, drawing the front foot back one-half step, and resumes a free-sparring stance.

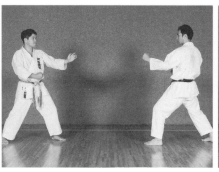

1

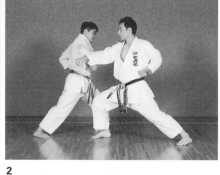

2

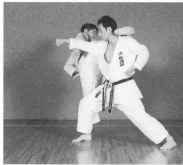

3

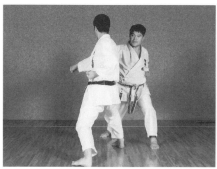

2'

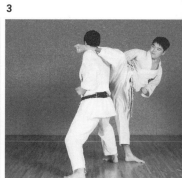

3'

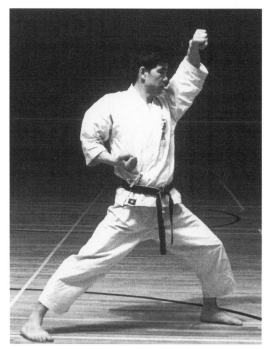

A rising block in front stance.

Chūdan Oi-Zuki No. 5

1. Attacker (right) and defender face off in free-sparring stance.

2. Stepping forward and to the outside with the front foot (left foot in photo), the defender blocks with *gyaku gedan-barai* (reverse downward block).

3. The defender then counters with *jōdan ushiro mawashi-geri* (upper-level back roundhouse kick).

4–5. Pulling the kicking leg to the rear, the defender sweeps the attacker's front leg (photos 4 & 5). Following the kick, the defender grabs the attacker's arm with the *uke-te* (blocking hand) and uses it to throw the attacker over when sweeping the leg.

6–7. After the throw, the defender deflects the attacker's arm with the edge of the left hand (photo 6) and follows through with a downward *gyaku-zuki* (photo 7).

8. The defender recovers, standing upright.

2'–8'. Side-angle views of photos 2 to 8.

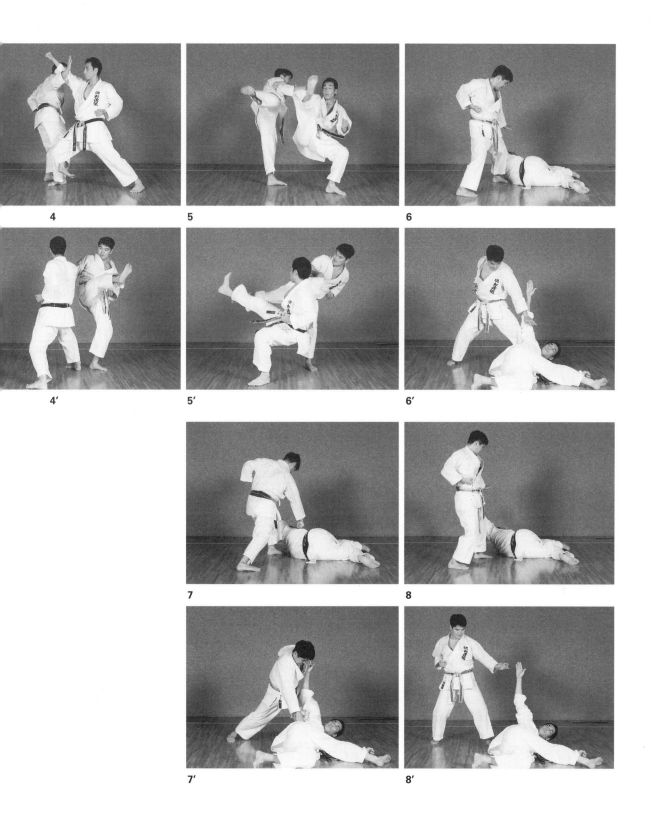

4 **5** **6**

4' **5'** **6'**

7 **8**

7' **8'**

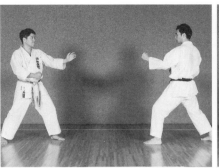 1

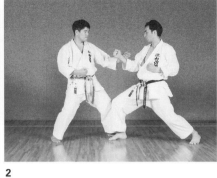 2

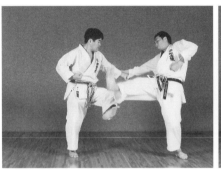 3

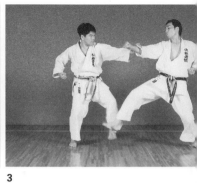 4

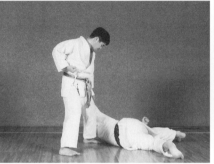 5

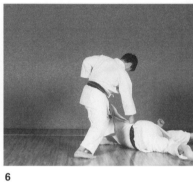 6

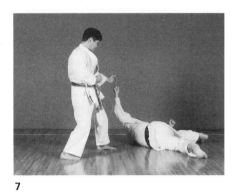 7

Chūdan Oi-Zuki No. 6

1. Attacker (right) and defender face off in free-sparring stance.

2–4. As the attacker commences his attack, the defender blocks with an open-handed *nagashi-uke* (sweeping block) while simultaneously sweeping the attacker's front leg with *ashi-barai* (leg sweep).

5–6. The defender counters with a downward *gyaku-zuki* (photo 6).

7. The defender recovers, standing upright.

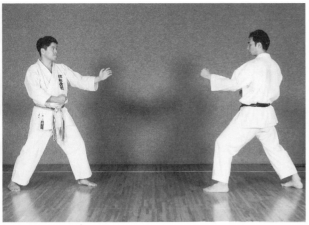

1

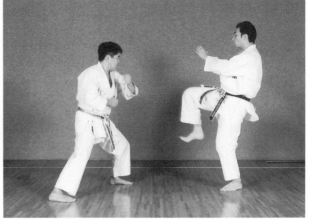

2

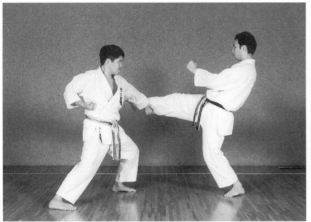

3

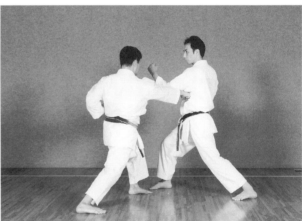

4

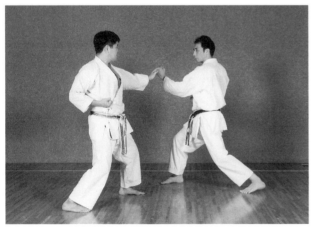

5

Mae-Geri (Front Snap Kick) No. 1

1. Attacker (right) and defender face off in free-sparring stance.

2–3. Pivoting on the front foot (left foot in photo), the defender shifts 45 degrees to the right while blocking with *gedan-barai* (downward block).

4. Utilizing the reaction from the block, the defender immediately counters with *chūdan gyaku-zuki* (middle-level reverse punch).

5. The defender recovers, retracting the *tsuki-te* (punching hand; right hand in photo) while simultaneously drawing the front foot (left foot in photo) back one-half step.

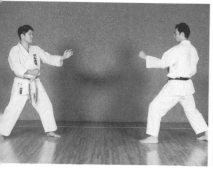 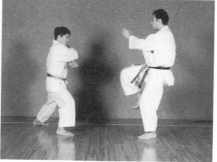 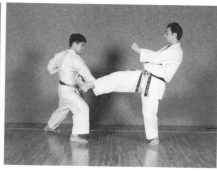

1

2

3

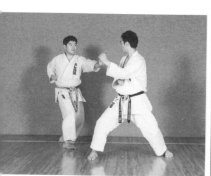 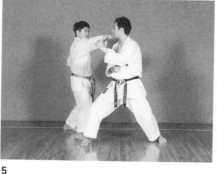 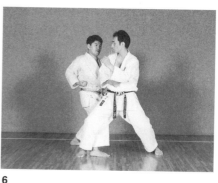

4

5

6

Mae-Geri No. 2

1. Attacker (right) and defender face off in free-sparring stance.

2–3. Pivoting on the rear foot (right foot in photo), the defender retracts the front foot to the left and rear at a 45-degree angle while blocking with *gedan-barai* in *zenkutsu-dachi* (front stance).

4. The defender draws the front foot back one-half step while simultaneously pulling the blocking hand (right hand in photo) back to the hip and thrusting the other hand forward in *tate shutō* (vertical knife-hand). The front foot is drawn back by utilizing the bending of the knee of the rear leg.

5. Thrusting off the back foot, the defender immediately counters with *choku-zuki* (straight punch), stepping behind the attacker's front foot.

6. Following the counterattack, the defender draws close to the attacker (enabling the defender to easily employ a throwing technique at any time).

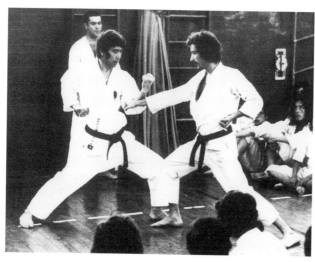

At a 1974 training session in Portugal.

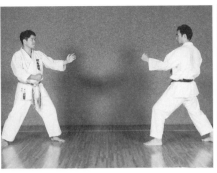
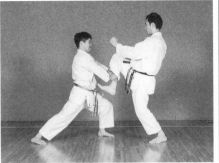
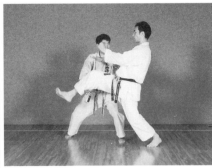

1 **2** **3**

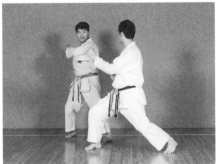

4 **5**

Mae-Geri No. 3

1. Attacker (right) and defender face off in free-sparring stance.

2. As the attacker commences his attack, the defender steps forward with the front foot (left foot in photo), blocking with *gedan jūji-uke* (lower-level X-block) (with the left hand above the right). When performing the *jūji-uke*, the distribution of blocking force between the right and left arms is 70% and 30%, respectively.

3. Utilizing the impact of the kick, the defender sweeps the attacker's kicking leg past using the right arm while shifting the back foot (right foot in photo) to the rear and left at a 45-degree angle.

4. While rotating the body (*tenshin*), the defender simultaneously counters with *jōdan shutō-uchi* (upper-level knife-hand strike).

5. The defender pulls back the striking hand while drawing the front foot back one-half step.

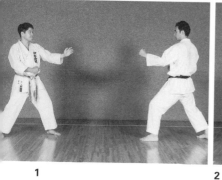
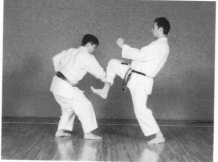
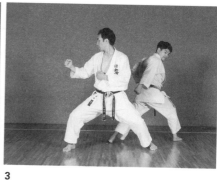

1

2

3

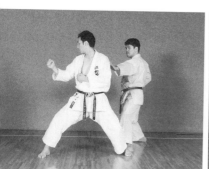
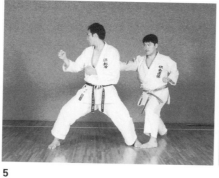
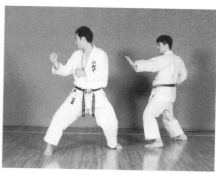

4

5

6

Mae-Geri No. 4

1. Attacker (right) and defender face off in free-sparring stance.

2–3. As the attacker moves in, the defender takes a large step forward and past the defender to the left. Halfway through the step, the defender blocks with *osae-uke* (pressing block) (photo 2), which then becomes *nagashi-uke* (sweeping block) (photo 3).

4–5. Pivoting on the front foot (right foot in photo), the defender immediately turns 180 degrees counterclockwise (photo 4) and counters with *chūdan gyaku-zuki* (photo 5).

6. When retracting the *tsuki-te* (punching hand; right hand in photo), the defender simultaneously draws the front foot back one-half step.

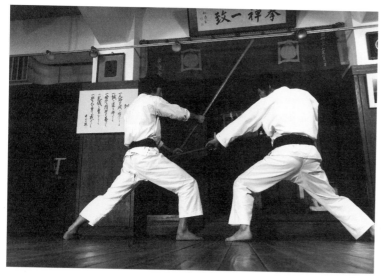

Delivering a back-fist strike at the Hōitsugan Dōjō.

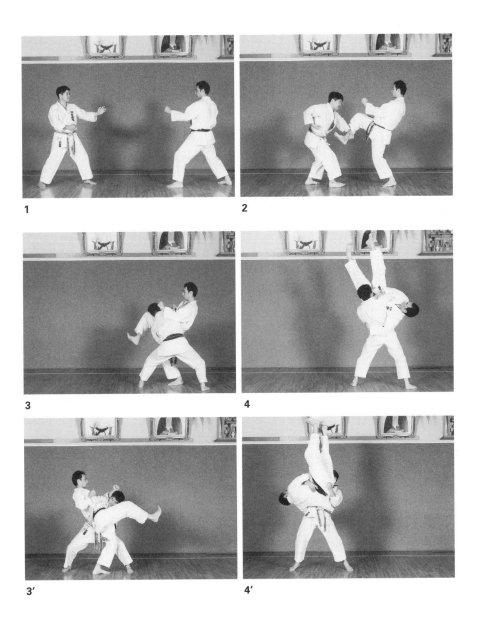

Mae-Geri No. 5

1. Attacker (right) and defender face off in free-sparring stance.

2. As the attacker approaches, the defender steps forward blocking with *gedan gyaku osae-uke* (lower-level reverse pressing block). The block is performed three-quarters of the way through the step.

3. During the remaining quarter-step forward, the defender places the *uke-te* (blocking hand; left hand in photo) behind the attacker's supporting leg and assumes *kiba-dachi* (straddle-leg stance). The defender's other arm reaches across the attacker's abdomen.

4. The defender, lifting the attacker's supporting leg, uses the lower abdomen to hoist the attacker into an inverted position, from which he can be dropped. Great care must be taken when practicing this technique to prevent injury.

3'–4'. Reverse-angle views of photo 3 and 4.

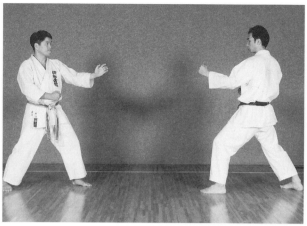

1

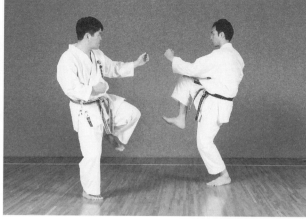

2

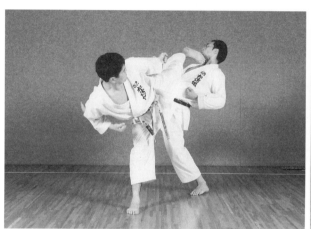

3

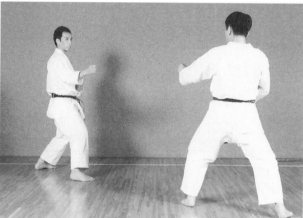

4

Mae-Geri No. 6

1. Attacker (right) and defender face off in free-sparring stance.

2–3. As the attacker approaches, the defender steps to the side with the back foot (right foot in photo), shifting his body out of the path of the attacker's kick (photo 2), and counters with *jōdan kekomi* (upper-level thrust kick) (photo 3).

4. The defender steps through and turns to once again face the attacker in free-sparring stance.

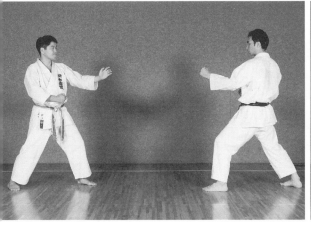

1

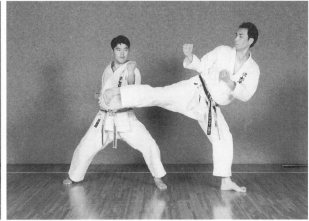

2

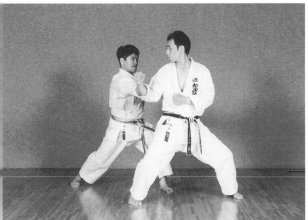

3

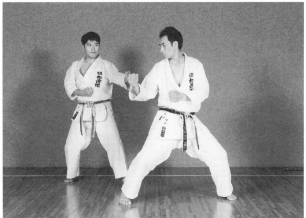

4

Yoko-Kekomi (Side Thrust Kick) No. 1

1. Attacker (right) and defender face off in free-sparring stance.

2. Pivoting on the front foot (left foot in photo), the defender shifts 45 degrees to the left while blocking with *chūdan soto ude-uke* (middle-level outside-to-inside block).

3. Utilizing the reaction from the block, the defender immediately counters with *chūdan gyaku-zuki* (middle-level reverse punch).

4. Following the counterattack, the defender, maintaining *zanshin* (physical and mental preparedness), recovers by drawing the front foot back one-half step while deflecting the attacker's arm with the blocking hand.

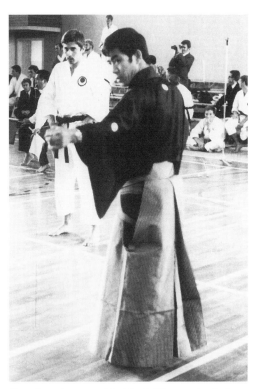

The author referees a match at the first European karate championship tournament.

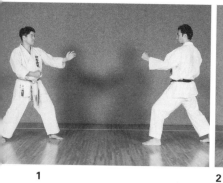 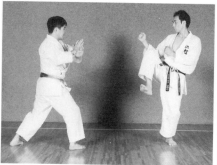 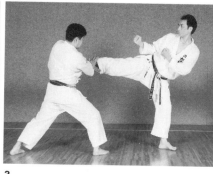

1
2
3

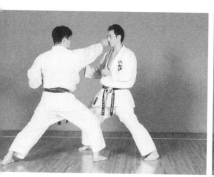 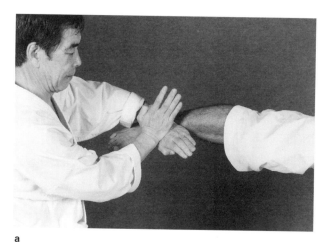

4
5

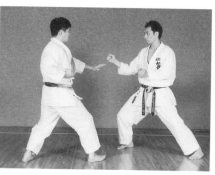

a

Yoko-Kekomi No. 2

1. Attacker (right) and defender face off in free-sparring stance.

2–3. Pivoting on the back foot (right foot in photo), the defender retracts the front foot back and to the right at a 45-degree angle while blocking with *awase* (two-handed) *seiryūtō-uke* (ox-jaw block). When blocking, the right hand is positioned above the wrist of the left (blocking) hand with the fingers pointed at the defender's face.

4. The defender counters with *tate-zuki* (vertical-fist punch) to the attacker's nose, utilizing the knee of the rear leg and the elbow of the right arm as springs to propel the lunge forward.

5. The defender pulls back the *tsuki-te* (punching hand; right hand in photo) sharply to the hip while simultaneously drawing the front foot back one-half step.

a. Close-up view of hand position for *awase seiryūtō-uke*.

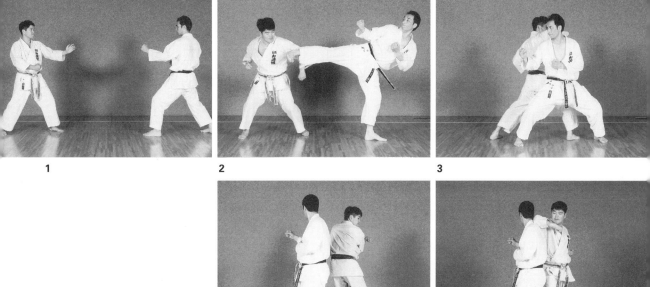

1   2   3

2'   3'

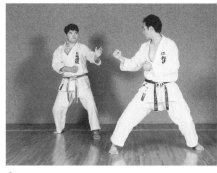

4

Yoko-Kekomi No. 3

1. Attacker (right) and defender face off in free-sparring stance.

2. The defender blocks with *haiwan-uke* (back-arm block).

3. Continuing with the motion that began with the block, the defender draws the front foot (left foot in photo) back one-half step and, pivoting on the same foot, swiftly turns 180 degrees, moving forward into *zenkutsu-dachi* (front stance) while simultaneously countering with *ushiro mawashi empi-uchi* (back roundhouse elbow strike). The transition from the block to the elbow strike should be a single flowing action with no unnecessary movements.

4. The defender recovers, pivoting on the same foot but turning in the opposite direction, and faces the attacker in free-sparring position.

2'. Side-angle view of defender immediately following block (between photos 2 and 3).

3'. Side-angle view of photo 3.

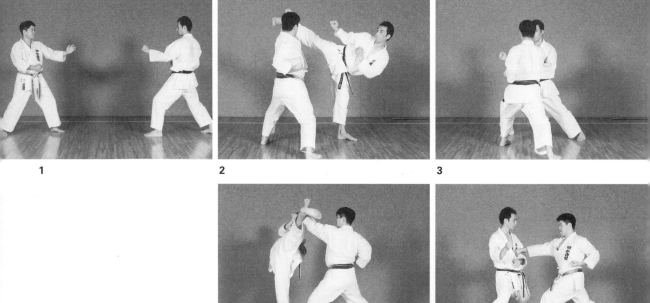

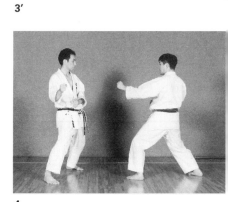

Mawashi-Geri (Roundhouse Kick) No. 1

1. Attacker (right) and defender face off in free-sparring stance.

2. Pivoting on the front foot (left foot in photo), the defender draws the back foot directly out to the side, turning 90 degrees while simultaneously blocking with *jōdan haiwan-uke* (upper-level back-arm block).

3. The defender counters with *chūdan gyaku-zuki* (middle-level reverse punch).

4. The defender recovers and resumes a free-sparring stance.

2'–3'. Side-angle views of photos 2 and 3.

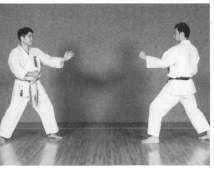
1

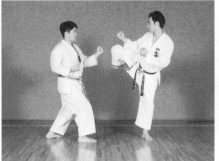
2

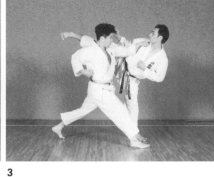
3

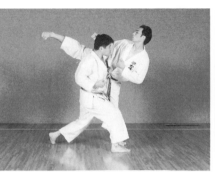
4

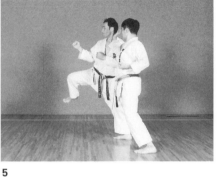
5

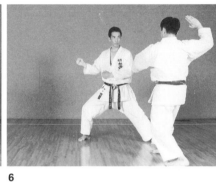
6

Mawashi-Geri No. 2

1. Attacker (right) and defender face off in free-sparring stance.

2–3. As the attacker approaches, the defender lunges forward (photo 2) and counters with *gyaku oi-zuki* (reverse lunge punch).

4–5. Following the punch (photo 4), the defender, pivoting on the front foot (right foot in photo), draws the back foot out to the side and turns 90 degrees while simultaneously striking with *shutō-uchi* (knife-hand strike) (photo 5).

6. The defender recovers, drawing the front foot back one-half step while pulling back the striking hand (*uchi-te*) and extending the pulling hand (*hiki-te*).

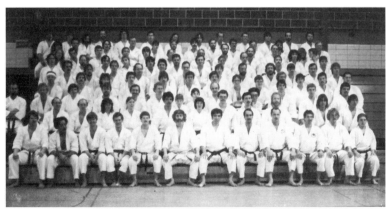

At the KUGB's first all-England training camp, held at the Alexander Palace circa 1969.

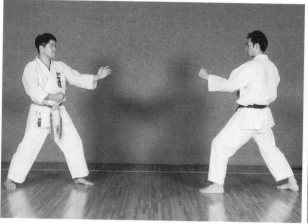

1

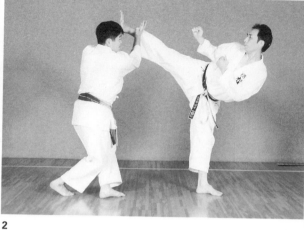

2

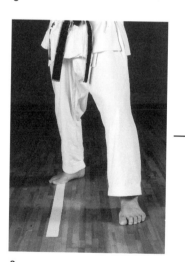

3

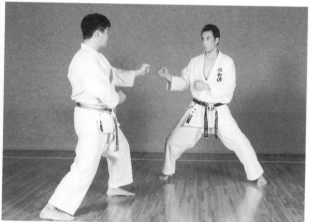

4

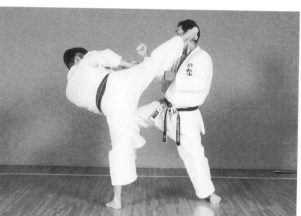

a → **b**

Mawashi-Geri No. 3

1. Attacker (right) and defender face off in free-sparring stance.

2. The defender draws the front foot (left foot in photo) back one-half step into *hiza kakushi-dachi* (hidden-knee stance), rotating the hips to the opposite side while blocking with *jōdan heikō-uke* (upper-level parallel block).

3. The defender immediately counters with *jōdan mawashi-geri*.

4. The defender recovers and assumes a free-sparring stance.

a–b. Close-up view of *hiza kakushi-dachi*.

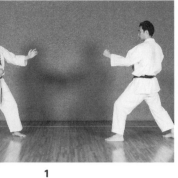 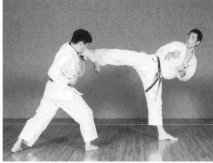 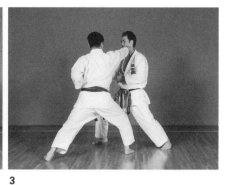

1   2   3

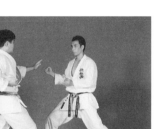 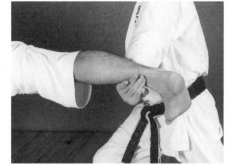 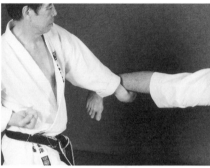

4   a   b

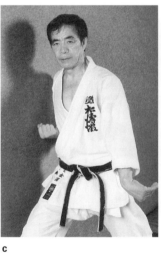 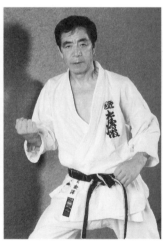 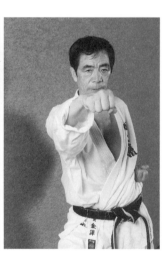

c   d   e

Ushiro-Geri (Back Kick) No. 1

1. Attacker (right) and defender face off in free-sparring stance.

2. Pivoting on the back foot (right foot in photo), the defender steps back and to the right with the front foot, shifting his body out of the path of the kick at a 45-degree angle while blocking with *gyaku sukui-uke* (reverse scooping block).

3. The defender immediately counters with *mawashi-zuki* (roundhouse punch).

4. The defender pulls back the *tsuki-te* (punching hand; right hand in photo) sharply to the hip while simultaneously drawing the front foot back one-half step.

a–b. Close-up views of *gyaku sukui-uke*.

c–e. Close-up view of *mawashi-zuki* following block. When executing the punch, the elbow should stay tucked in, traveling along the side of the body.

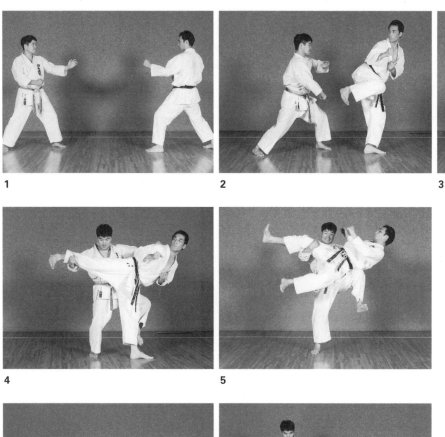

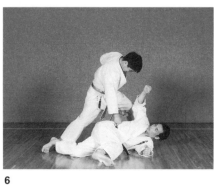
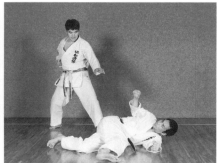

Ushiro-Geri No. 2

1. Attacker (right) and defender face off in free-sparring stance.

2–3. As the attacker commences his attack, the defender lunges forward (photo 2), positioning the front foot (left foot in photo) alongside the attacker's supporting leg while blocking with *sukui-uke* (scooping block) in *kiba-dachi* (straddle-leg stance) (photo 3).

4–5. With the blocking hand under the attacker's kicking leg, the defender sweeps the supporting leg with *ashi-barai* (leg sweep) (photo 4), lifting and dropping the attacker to the floor (photo 5).

6. The defender counters with a downward *gyaku-zuki* (reverse punch).

7. The defender recovers, standing upright.

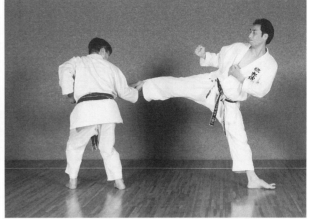

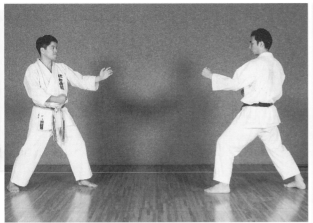

1

2

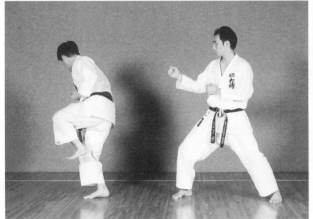

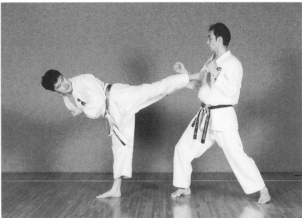

3

4

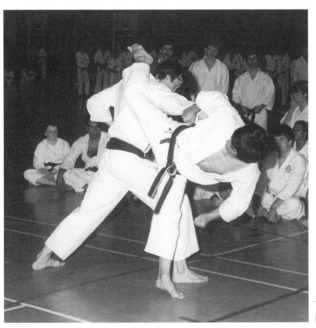

Ushiro-Geri No. 3

1. Attacker (right) and defender face off in free-sparring stance.

2. Pivoting on the back foot (right foot in photo), the defender draws the front foot to the rear while blocking with *sukui-uke*.

3–4. Continuing to turn in the same direction (photo 3), the defender immediately counters with *ushiro-geri* (photo 4).

The author demonstrates an upper-level back round-house kick during a training session in England.

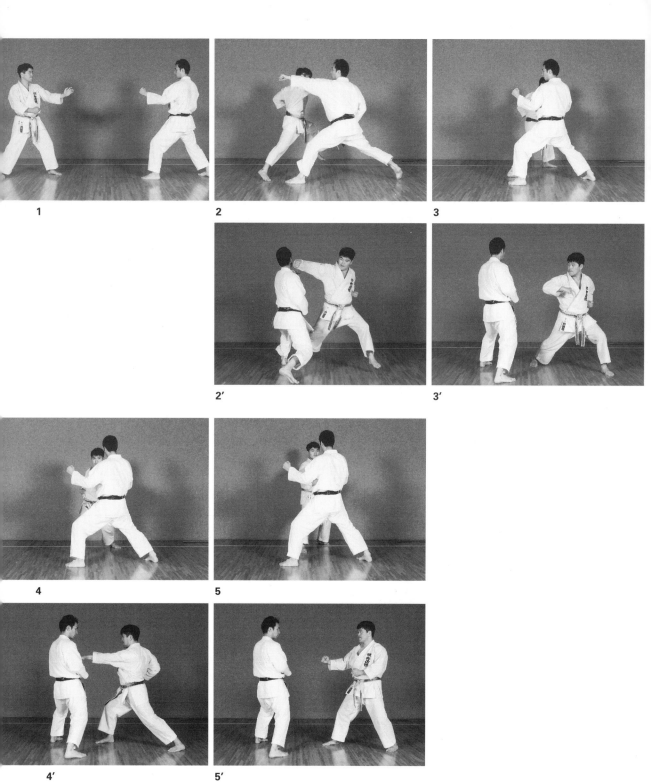

1

2

3

2′

3′

4

5

4′

5′

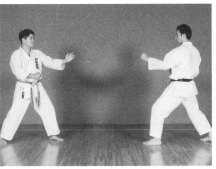

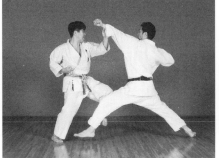

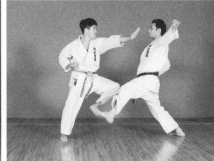

1 **2** **3**

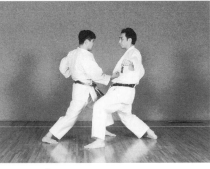

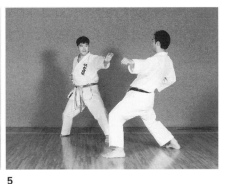

4 **5**

Jōdan Kizami-Zuki (Upper-Level Jab) No. 1 (left page)

1. Attacker (right) and defender face off in free-sparring stance.

2–3. As the attacker approaches, the defender steps outward at a 45-degree angle, thrusting off the back foot (right foot in photo) while striking with *jōdan uraken-uchi* (upper-level back-fist strike) (photo 2) into *zenkutsu-dachi* (front stance) (photo 3).

4. The defender immediately rotates the hips toward the attacker into *zenkutsu-dachi* while delivering *gyaku-zuki* (reverse punch).

5. The defender recovers and assumes a free-sparring stance.

2′–5′. Side-angle views of photos 2–5.

Jōdan Kizami-Zuki No. 2

1. Attacker (right) and defender face off in free-sparring stance.

2–3. The defender deflects the jab with *hirate-barai* (open-hand sweeping block) while simultaneously sweeping the attacker's front leg using *ashi-barai* (leg sweep).

4. The defender counters with *chūdan ura gyaku-zuki* (middle-level close reverse punch) at the instant that the attacker's front leg touches the floor.

5. Immediately following the counterattack, the defender thrusts the attacker away using the palm-heel of the hand against the shoulder and, pivoting on the front foot (left foot in photo), shifts away from the attacker at a 45-degree angle.

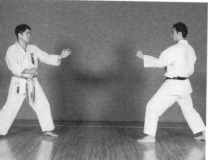

1

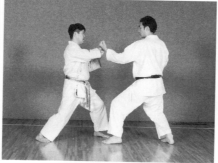

2

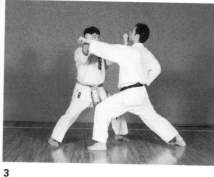

3

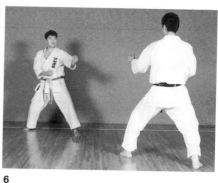

3'

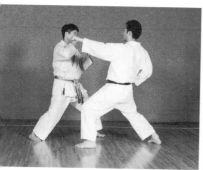

4

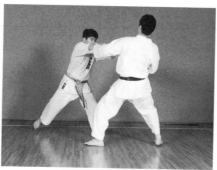

5

6

Jōdan Kizami-Zuki No. 3

1. Attacker (right) and defender face off in free-sparring stance.

2–3. As the attacker approaches, the defender lunges forward off the back foot, blocking with *haiwan nagashi-uke* (back-arm sweeping block) while simultaneously countering with *uraken-uchi* in *fudō-dachi* (rooted stance).

4–5. Following the counterattack, the defender thrusts the attacker back with both hands while shifting to the rear at a 45-degree angle.

6. The defender recovers and assumes a free-sparring stance.

3'. Side-angle view of photo 3.

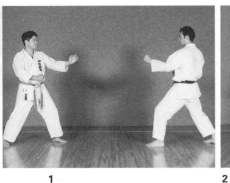
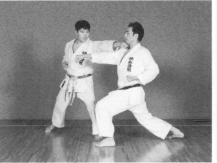
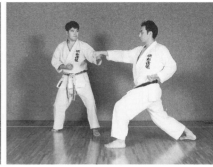

1 **2** **3**

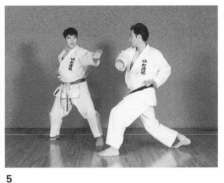

4 **5**

Chūdan Gyaku-Zuki (Middle-Level Reverse Punch) No. 1

1. Attacker (right) and defender face off in free-sparring stance.

2. Pivoting on the front foot (left foot in photo), the defender shifts 45 degrees to the left while countering with *jōdan kizami-zuki* (upper-level jab).

3. The defender immediately draws the elbow back toward the hip following the punch.

4. The defender follows through with *chūdan gyaku-zuki* (middle-level reverse punch).

5. When retracting the *tsuki-te* (punching hand; right hand in photo), the defender simultaneously draws the front foot back one-half step while deflecting the attacker's arm with the opposite hand.

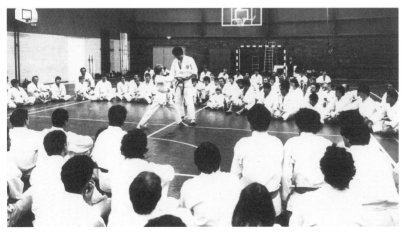

Explaining the correct way to execute a reverse punch.

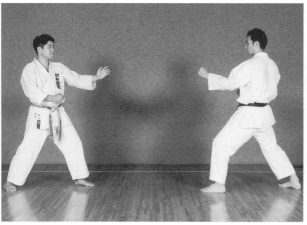

1

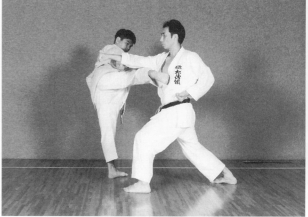

2

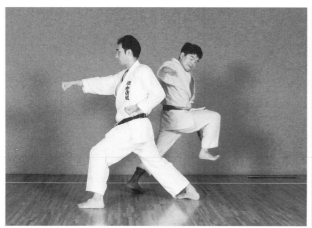

3

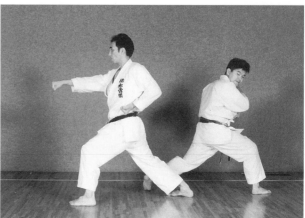

4

Chūdan Gyaku-Zuki No. 2

1. Attacker (right) and defender face off in free-sparring stance.

2. As the attacker approaches, the defender steps forward and out of the path of the punch, blocking with *gedan-barai* (downward block) while simultaneously countering with *chūdan mawashi-geri* (middle-level roundhouse kick).

3. As the second half of a continuous motion, the defender thrusts forward off the supporting leg (left leg in photo) while executing *ushiro shutō-uchi* (back knife-hand strike) to the back of the attacker's neck.

4. The defender follows through, pulling back the striking hand.

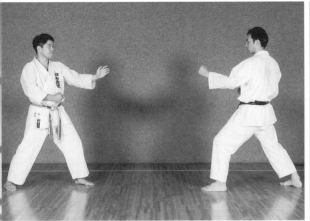

1

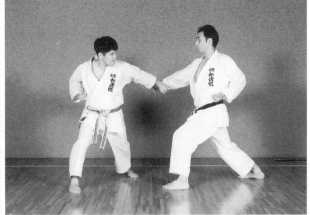

2

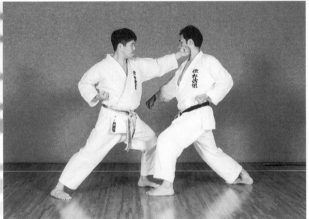

3

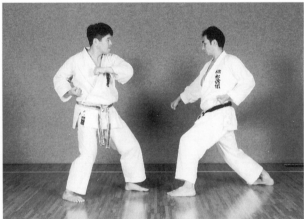

4

Chūdan Gyaku-Zuki No. 3

1. Attacker (right) and defender face off in free-sparring stance.

2. The defender steps out directly to the side with the back foot (right foot in photo) while blocking with *gedan-barai*.

3. Utilizing the force generated by thrusting off the front foot (right foot in photo), the defender, using the blocking hand, counters with *uraken-uchi* (back-fist strike).

4. The defender pulls back the striking hand while drawing the front foot back one-half step.

OKURI JIYŪ IPPON-KUMITE (Follow-Through Free-Style One-Step Kumite)

Okuri jiyū ippon-kumite (follow-through free-style one-step *kumite*) begins in the same manner as *jiyū ippon kumite*, but after the initial attack, the attacker freely launches a second assault without pre-announcing the intended target or technique that will be used. The defender, after completing his first counterattack, must immediately ready mind and body in preparation for the follow-up attack. In response to the second attack, the defender must also finish with a counterattack.

In *kumite*, even if an attacker were to deliver a blow with the speed and force to fell an opponent, should the opponent have the strength to withstand the attack, it would be difficult to decide the bout with a single strike. Accordingly, a second attack would be called for.

The same principle applies in defensive circumstances. Even if an attack were effectively blocked or evaded and a counterattack launched, there would be no assurance that the effort would be sufficient to stop the opponent. As such, it is essential that the defender maintain ample composure and preparedness after an initial attack to deal effectively with any subsequent assaults.

This is why, with regard to continuous offensive and defensive sequences, it is necessary to strive for improved mental, technical, and physical abilities. Training thoroughly to sharpen reflexes, increase speed, and develop physical, mental, and breathing control fosters techniques that maintain their integrity, even when performed in succession.

Okuri jiyū ippon-kumite was designed as the ideal training method to achieve these objectives. The attacker, beginning from a free-sparring stance, announces the target and the technique to follow before launching an attack with speed and power, paying careful attention to timing in an attempt to catch the defender off-guard. The attacker may employ such techniques as feints and false starts to confuse the defender, throw off his timing, or catch him off-balance as a means of further enhancing the training process.

The defender must pay close attention to the attacker, waiting patiently for the attack without being tricked or intimidated. The defender must also maintain the peace of mind to tell whether his opponent is launching a genuine attack or merely a feint with the aim of creating an opportunity. When the first attack is judged to be real, the defender responds as he would in *jiyū ippon kumite*, moving in one of the eight possible directions, blocking or avoiding the technique while responding with a counterattack.

At the moment the attacker has confirmed that the defender's counterattack has concluded, he must instantaneously assess the location of his opponent, specifically the direction and distance (*maai*), and then launch a forceful and effective second attack at will.

The defender must possess a fighting spirit that does not succumb to that of the attacker. While maintaining the same level of earnest intensity that would be called for if confronting knives instead of fists and feet, the defender must wait calmly for the second attack without fearing it or acting in haste. Carefully assessing his opponent's strike or kick, watching it until it almost reaches the intended target, the defender then immediately responds. He may either shift his body while blocking and then counterattack, or shift out of the path of the attack while simultaneously countering. After the counterattack, the defender resumes a free-sparring stance.

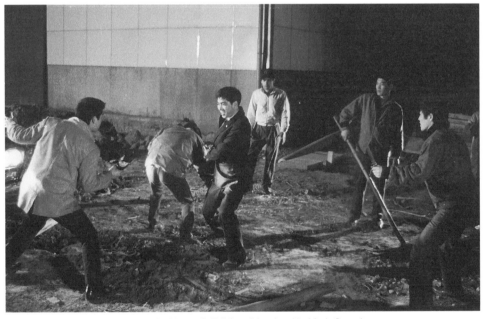

A snapshot from the filming of the movie "Karate: Self-defense" (produced by Movie Center).

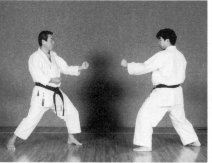

1

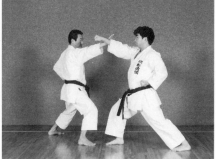

2

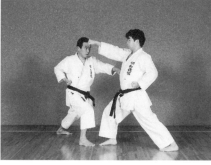

3

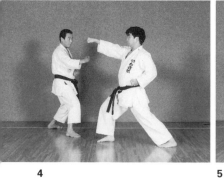

4

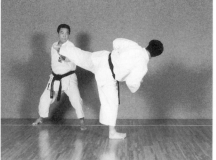

5

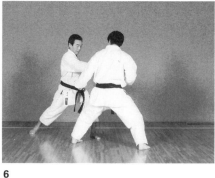

6

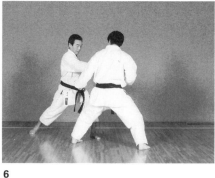

7

Okuri Jiyū Ippon-Kumite No. 1

1. Attacker (right) and defender face off.
2. Attacker delivers *jōdan oi-zuki* (upper-level lunge punch). / Defender steps back at 45-degree angle and blocks with *jōdan harai-uke* (upper-level sweeping block).
3. Defender counters with *chūdan gyaku-zuki* (middle-level reverse punch).
4. Defender recovers.
5. Attacker delivers *kekomi* (thrust kick). / Defender steps back and blocks with *soto ude-uke* (outside-to-inside block).
6. Defender counters with *chūdan gyaku-zuki*.
7. Attacker and defender recover.

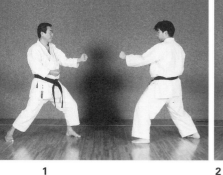

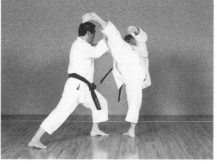

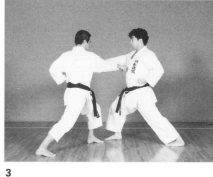

1

2

3

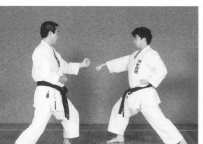

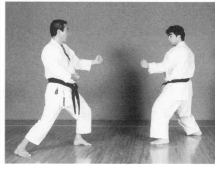

4

5

6

Okuri Jiyū Ippon-Kumite No. 2

1. Attacker (right) and defender face off.
2. Attacker delivers *chūdan oi-zuki*. / Defender shifts 45 degrees and blocks with *gedan-barai* (downward block).
3. Defender counters with *chūdan gyaku-zuki*.
4. Defender recovers.
5. Attacker delivers *jōdan mawashi-geri* (upper-level roundhouse kick). / Defender blocks with *haiwan-uke* (back-arm block) while simultaneously countering with *kizami-zuki* (jab).
6. Attacker and defender recover.

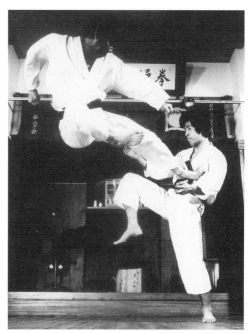

Performing a flying kick at the Hōitsugan Dōjō.

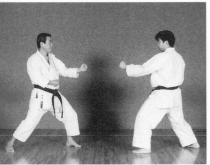

1

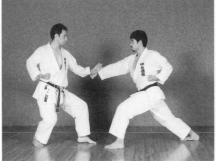

2

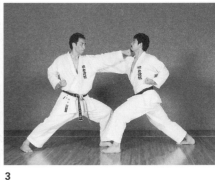

3

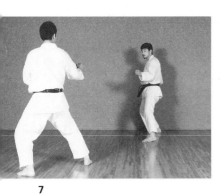

4

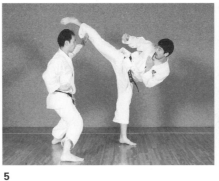

5

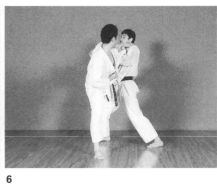

6

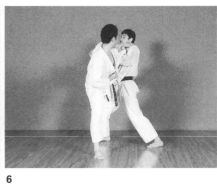

7

Okuri Jiyū Ippon-Kumite No. 3

1. Attacker (right) and defender face off.
2. Attacker delivers *chūdan gyaku-zuki.* / Defender takes half-step back and blocks with *seiryūtō-uke* (ox-jaw block).
3. Defender thrusts off back foot and counters with *kizami-zuki.*
4. Attacker and defender recover.
5. Attacker delivers *jōdan mawashi-geri.* / Defender steps out to side with back foot and blocks with *tate shutō-uke* (vertical knife-hand block).
6. Defender draws back foot in to close distance to attacker and counters with *kizami yoko-geri* (short side kick).
7. Attacker and defender recover.

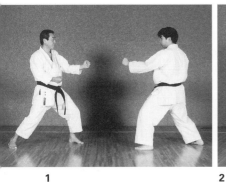

1

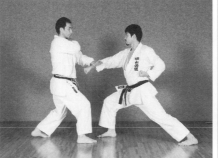

2

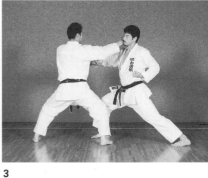

3

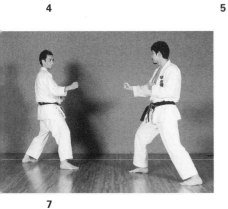

4

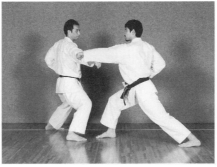

5

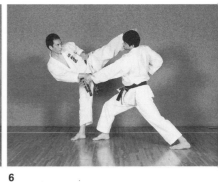

6

7

Okuri Jiyū Ippon-Kumite No. 4

1. Attacker (right) and defender face off.
2. Attacker delivers *chūdan oi-zuki*. / Defender steps back and blocks with *osae-uke* (pressing block).
3. Defender thrusts off back foot and counters with *uraken-uchi* (back-fist strike).
4. Defender pulls back striking hand and draws front foot back one-half step.
5. Attacker delivers *gyaku-zuki*. / Defender shifts 45 degrees and blocks with *gedan-barai*.
6. Defender counters with *jōdan mawashi-geri*.
7. Attacker and defender recover.

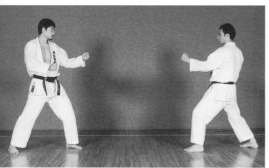

1

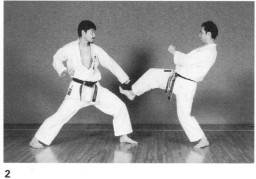

2

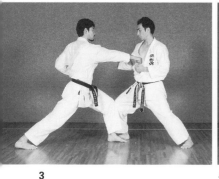

3

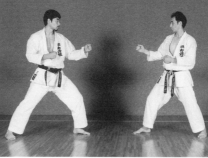

4

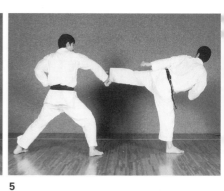

5

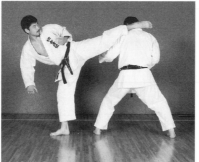

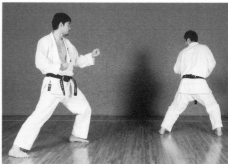

6

7

8

Okuri Jiyū Ippon-Kumite No. 5

1. Attacker (right) and defender face off.
2. Attacker delivers *mae-geri* (front snap kick). / Defender blocks with *gedan-barai*.
3. Defender counters with *gyaku-zuki*.
4. Attacker and defender recover.
5. Attacker delivers *yoko-geri kekomi* (side thrust kick). / Defender steps back and blocks with *haiwan-uke*.
6. Defender draws front foot back one-half step in preparation for counterattack.
7. Defender counters with *jōdan ushiro mawashi-geri* (upper-level back roundhouse kick).
8. Defender recovers.

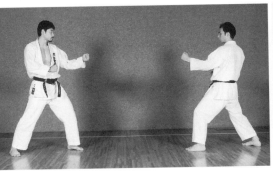
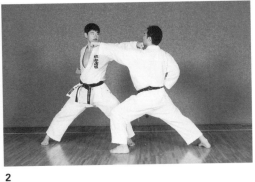

1

2

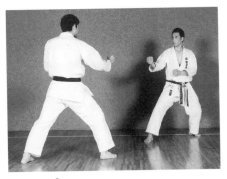
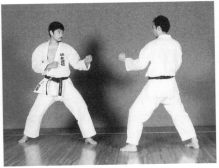
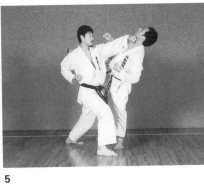

3

4

5

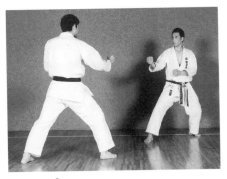

6

Okuri Jiyū Ippon-Kumite No. 6

1. Attacker (right) and defender face off.
2. Attacker delivers *jōdan kizami-zuki*. / Defender utilizes body rotation to shift out of the path of the attack while simultaneously executing *jōdan kizami-zuki*.
3. Defender follows through with *gyaku-zuki*.
4. Attacker and defender recover.
5. As attacker commences *mawashi-geri* attack, defender lunges forward with *jōdan gyaku-zuki*.
6. Attacker and defender recover.

JIYŪ KUMITE (Free Sparring Kumite)

Jiyū kumite (free sparring) provides karate practitioners with the opportunity to freely apply the offensive and defensive techniques—punches, kicks, strikes, and blocks—that they have trained hard to develop. In *jiyū kumite*, neither attacks nor intended targets are prearranged and both opponents fully utilize their strength, spirit, and skill.

When engaging in *jiyū kumite*, both participants must suppose a contest of life-or-death consequences, achieving a combat-ready state of mind enabling each to embrace the challenge of the duel.

The *jiyū kumite* matches that have become a popular fixture of karate tournaments today are carried out in accordance with competition regulations. The contestants must show respect toward each other while maintaining a level of dignity that is worthy of such respect. They also bear the heavy responsibility and trust that is essential when exchanging blows of deadly force, halting their strikes at a point just before they make contact with the intended target. Tactics employed in competition include carefully reading an opponent's breathing, emotions and *maai* (distance between opponents).

The main objective of sports-oriented karate is to gain victory over one's opponent. The main objective of karate as a martial art is to triumph over one's self. It is important to fully appreciate this distinction when seeking victory in competitive karate.

MATCH-STYLE KUMITE VS. TOURNAMENT KUMITE

Match-style kumite

While there are no competitive encounters in karate as a martial art, match-style (*shiai*) *kumite* provides a substitute for actual combat that enables practitioners to experience firsthand an authentic exchange of offensive and defensive techniques. Match-style *kumite* represents a means of testing skills and abilities to freely evaluate one's mental, physical, and technical prowess.

Unlike tournament *kumite*, match-style *kumite* does not adhere to any special rules, such as those stipulated in competition regulations. One's conscience dictates the only rules that exist for this type of *kumite* and, within the framework of these rules, practitioners call on the mental, physical, and technical faculties that they have developed and polished through daily training.

The *shiai-kumite* of karate-dō is characterized by attacks of deadly force that are controlled to stop a mere inch in front of their intended target.

Mastering the control of one's body and limbs facilitates the control of one's spirit, which fosters self-discipline and contributes to the building of character. Because there are no formal rules, the threat of serious injury poses a genuine risk. Accordingly, *shiai-kumite* relies heavily on not only the participants' sense of responsibility, but also on mutual trust.

The true essence of karate-dō boils down to how to control a strike that is powerful enough to kill with a single blow by delivering it so that its explosive force culminates at the instant before it reaches its target. This ability can only be achieved through the diligent and steady training of first *tanren* (training) *kumite*, followed by *kihon* (basic) *kumite*, and then *yakusoku* (promise) *kumite*.

Tournament kumite

Tournament *kumite* refers to competitive sparring matches that pit the mental, physical, and technical skills of contestants to determine a victor within the framework of competition and officiating regulations.

As the matches are presided over and decided by referees and judges, contestants must thoroughly study all related tournament regulations in addition to carrying out their usual training. Furthermore, the ability to swiftly evaluate a referee's personality and temperament, just as one would an opponent, is an important skill.

Although an extreme argument, compared with the deadly force and correct form of karate-dō as a martial art, unorthodox techniques that lack destructive power are more difficult to block. In addition, since such techniques do not pose much risk of injury in the event that contact is made, there is less chance that they would result in penalization.

This line of thinking may lead some to ask: "Then what is the point of spending time striking a *makiwara* (punching board) to develop techniques of deadly force if it is forbidden to make contact? Would it not make more sense to use that time training in other areas?"

Karate-dō is not merely a combative contest to determine victory or defeat. But, as competitions held in accordance with modern rules are now commonplace, it is only natural that participants in these events should seek to be victorious.

Accordingly, while this argument is an extreme example, in the case of tournament *kumite*, it is the extreme that could very well open the path to victory.

It should be pointed out that the above comment is intended for those karate practitioners who are concerned primarily with taking part in tournament-style competitions.

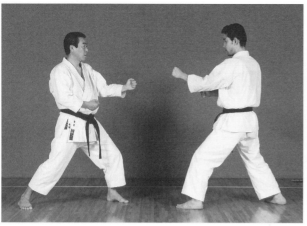

1

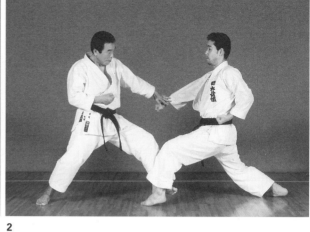

2

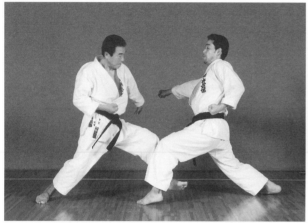

3

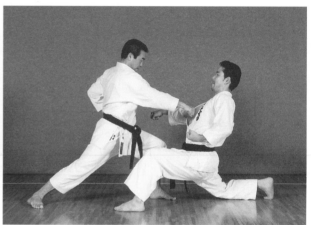

4

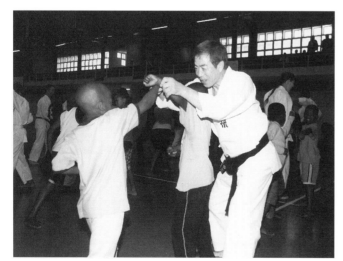

Teaching the correct way to execute a front punch to the street children in the Republic of South Africa in 2003.

Jiyū Kumite No. 1

1. Opponent A (left) and opponent B face off in free-sparring stance.

2–3. A deflects B's *chūdan gyaku-zuki* (middle-level reverse punch) (photo 2) while simultaneously sweeping B's front leg with *ashi-barai* (leg sweep) (photos 2 and 3).

4. A counters with *chūdan gyaku-zuki*.

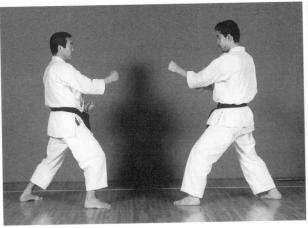

1

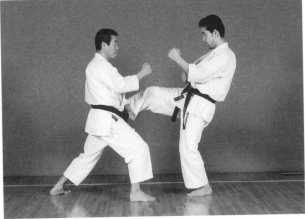

2

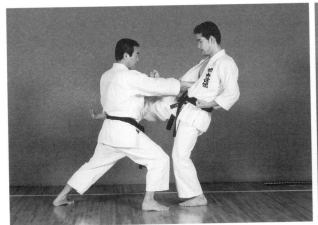

3

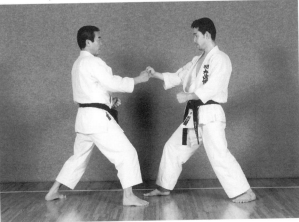

4

Jiyū Kumite No. 2

1. Opponent A (left) and opponent B face off in free-sparring stance.

2–3. A blocks B's *chūdan mae-geri* (middle-level front snap kick) with gyaku *gedan-barai* (reverse downward block) (photos 2 and 3) while simultaneously countering with *chūdan jun-zuki* (middle-level front punch) (photo 3).

4. A and B recover and resume free-sparring stances.

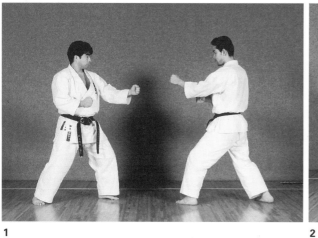

1

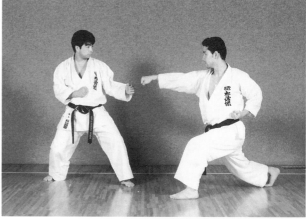

2

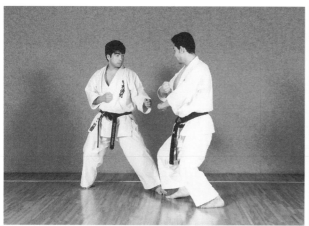

3

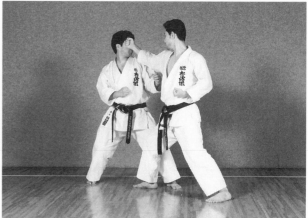

4

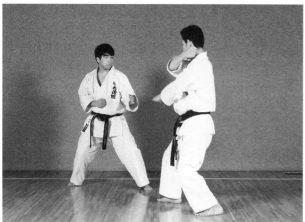

5

Jiyū Kumite No. 3

1. Opponent A (left) and opponent B face off in free-sparring stance.

2. Opponent A (left) turns at a 45-degree angle to opponent B as B delivers *chūdan gyaku-zuki*.

3. B draws the back foot forward and lunges toward A.

4. B executes *uraken-uchi* (back-fist strike) to A's temple.

5. B draws back the striking hand while distancing himself from A in anticipation of a possible counterattack.

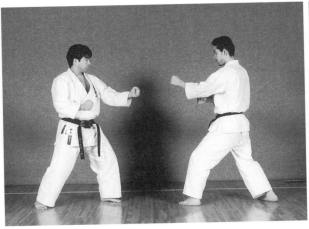

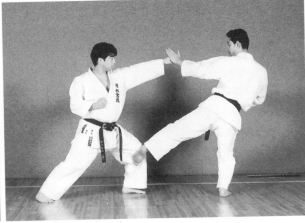

1 **2**

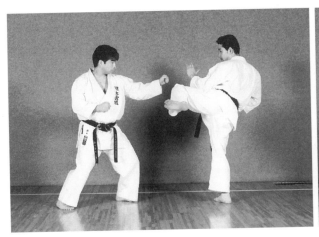

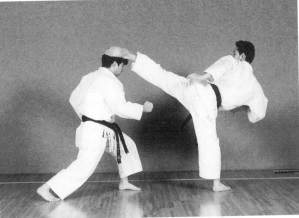

3 **4**

Jiyū Kumite No. 4

1. Opponent A (left) and opponent B face off in free-sparring stance.
2. B blocks A's *jōdan kizami-zuki* (upper-level jab) with *hirate-uke* (open-hand block) while simultaneously executing *gedan kizami mawashi-geri* (lower-level short roundhouse kick).
3-4. Adjusting the delivery to A's movement (photo 3), B counters with *jōdan kizami mawashi-geri*.

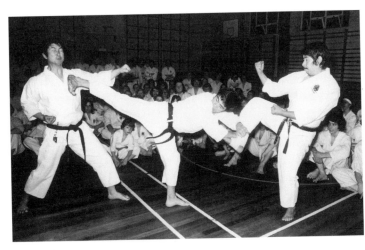

Demonstrating how to defend against two simultaneous attacks in England with Shirō Asano (left) and Sadashige Katō.

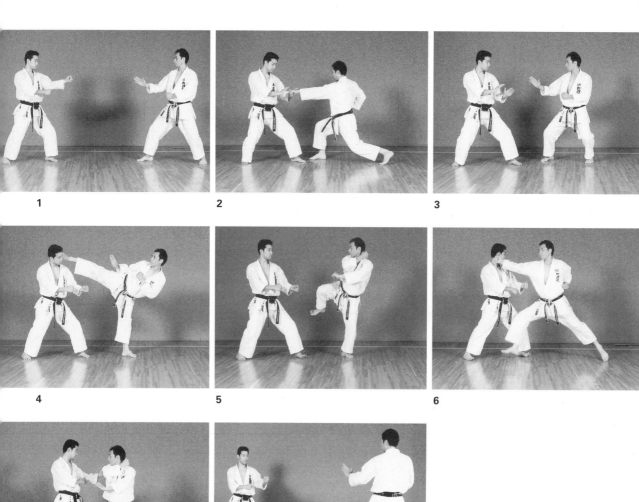

1 2 3

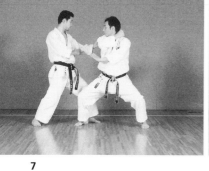

4 5 6

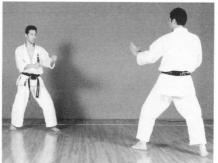

7 8

Jiyū Kumite No. 5

1. Opponent A (left) and opponent B face off in free-sparring stance.

2–3. Upon finding an opportunity, B delivers *chūdan gyaku-zuki* (photo 2) and closes the distance to A by drawing the back foot forward (photo 3).

4. B executes *kizami mawashi-geri*.

5–6. Upon withdrawing the kicking leg (photo 5), B immediately follows through with a lunging *uraken-uchi* (photo 6).

7–8. B withdraws the striking hand (photo 7) and immediately distances himself from A, resuming a free-sparring stance (photo 8).

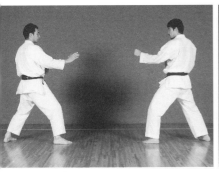 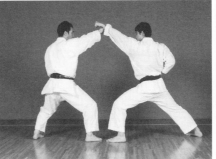 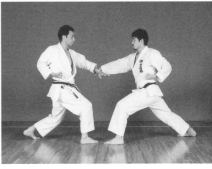

1 **2** **3**

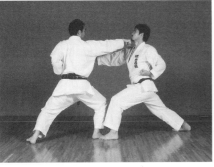 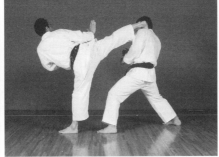 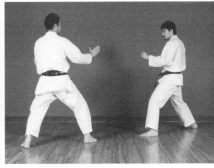

4 **5** **6**

Jiyū Kumite No. 6

1. Opponent A (left) and opponent B face off in free-sparring stance.
2. A blocks B's *kizami-zuki* with *jōdan shutō uke* (upper-level knife-hand block).
3. A blocks B's *chūdan gyaku-zuki* with *gyaku chūdan shutō-uke*.
4. A immediately counters with *kizami-zuki*.
5. A finishes off with *kizami mawashi-geri*.
6. A recovers and resumes a free-sparring stance.

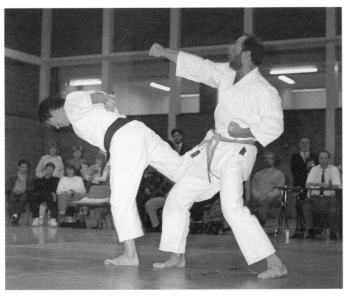

Demonstrating a back kick.

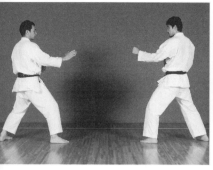 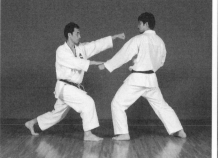 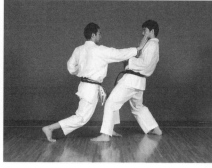

1   2   3

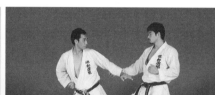 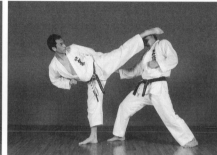

4   5   6

Jiyū Kumite No. 7

1. Opponent A (left) and opponent B face off in free-sparring stance.
2. A checks B with *jōdan gyaku-zuki* while restraining B's front hand.
3. While B leans backward, A moves forward and pushes B off balance.
4. A immediately follows through with *jun-zuki*.
5. A retracts the punching hand while simultaneously drawing the back foot forward.
6. A finishes off with *kizami ushiro mawashi-geri* (short back roundhouse kick)

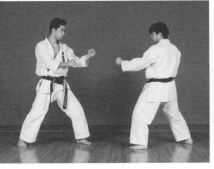

1

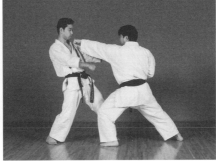

2

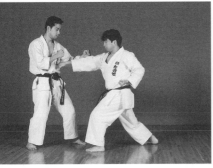

3

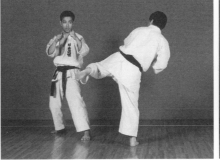

4

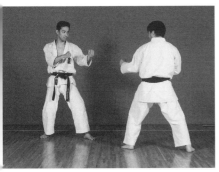

5

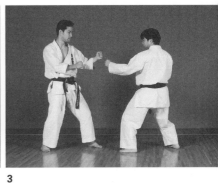

6

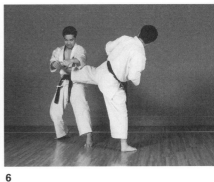

7

Jiyū Kumite No. 8

1. Opponent A (left) and opponent B face off in free-sparring stance.

2–4. B delivers *kizami-zuki* (photo 2) and immediately follows through with *chūdan gyaku-zuki* (photo 4).

5–6. While A retreats, B draws the back foot forward one-half step (photo 5) and finishes off with *chūdan kizami mawashi-geri* (photo 6).

7. B recovers and assumes a free-sparring stance.

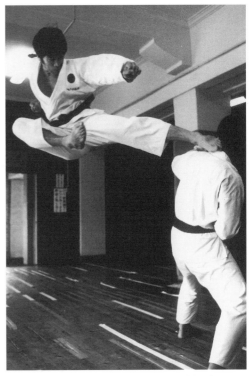

The author performs a flying kick at the JKA headquarters dōjō in Kōrakuen, Tokyo.

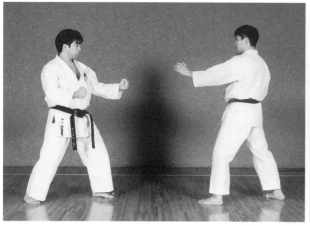

1

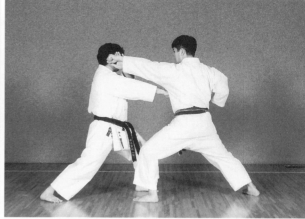

2

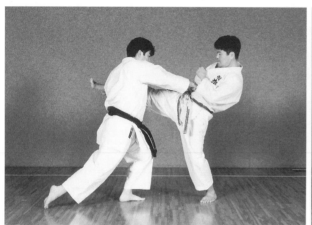

3

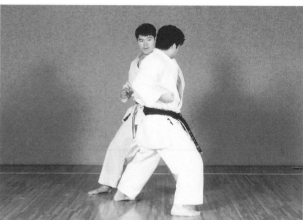

4

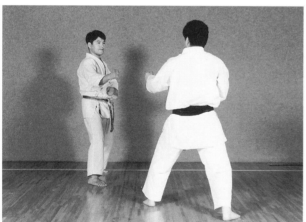

5

Jiyū Kumite No. 9

1. Opponent A (left) and opponent B face off in free-sparring stance.

2. A deflects B's *kizami-zuki* with *jōdan nagashi-uke* (upper-level sweeping block) while simultaneously countering with *chūdan gyaku-zuki*.

3. A blocks B's *mae-geri* with *gedan-barai* while simultaneously countering with *chūdan gyaku-zuki*.

4–5. A draws back the punching hand (photo 4), recovers, and assumes a free-sparring stance (photo 5).

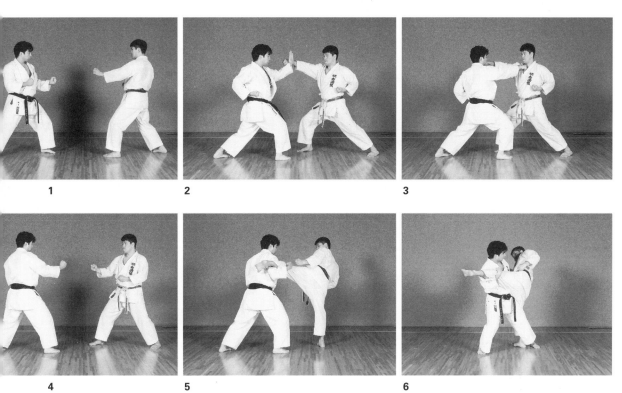

1

2

3

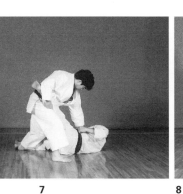

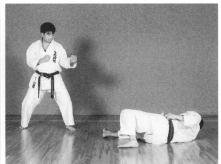

4

5

6

7

8

Jiyū Kumite No. 10

1. Opponent A (left) and opponent B face off in free-sparring stance.
2. A takes one step back and blocks B's *jōdan oi-zuki* (upper-level lunge punch) with *jōdan nagashi-uke*.
3. A immediately counters with *jōdan jun-zuki*.
4. A and B reestablish their *maai* (distance of separation) in anticipation of a follow-up exchange.
5. A evades B's *chūdan mawashi-geri* while catching B's kicking leg.
6. A uses the back foot to sweep B's supporting leg.
7. After throwing B to the floor, A finishes off with *gyaku-zuki*.
8. A recovers and assumes a free-sparring stance.

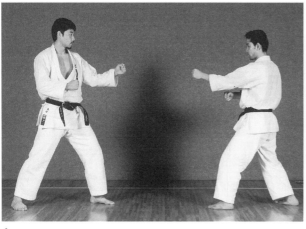

1

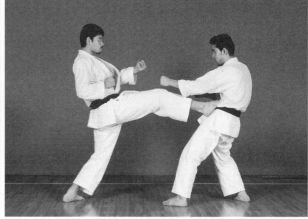

2

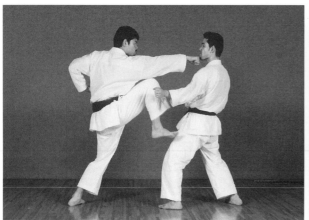

3

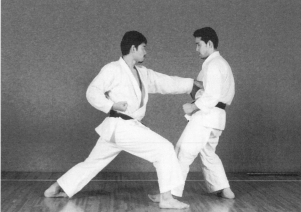

4

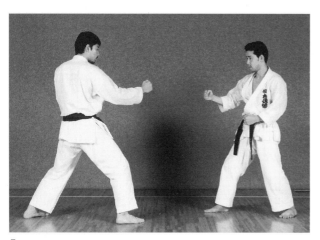

5

Jiyū Kumite No. 11

1. Opponent A (left) and opponent B face off in free-sparring stance.

2. A delivers *chūdan mae-geri*.

3. A follows through with *jōdan kizami-zuki* immediately upon retracting the kicking foot.

4. At the instant that A's kicking foot touches the floor, he finishes off with *chūdan gyaku-zuki*.

5. A recovers and assumes a free-sparring stance.

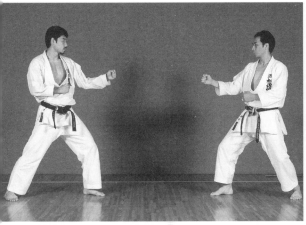

1

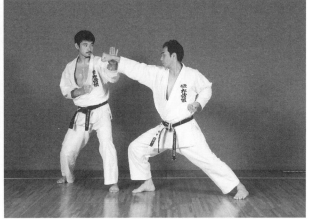

2

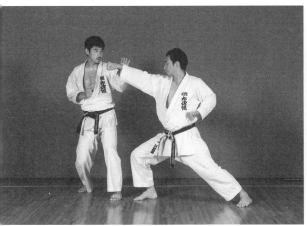

3

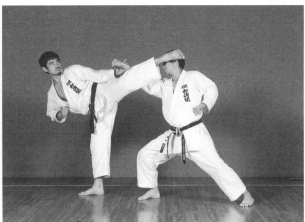

4

Jiyū Kumite No. 12

1. Opponent A (left) and opponent B face off in free-sparring stance.

2. A, pivoting on the front foot, shifts 90 degrees out of the path of B's *jōdan kizami-zuki* while blocking with *hirate-uke*.

3–4. A draws his back foot forward one-half step (photo 3) and counters with *kizami ushiro mawashi-geri*.

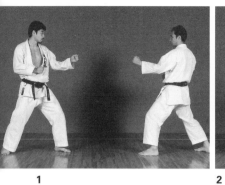

1

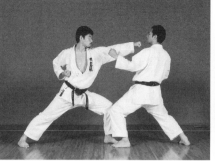

2

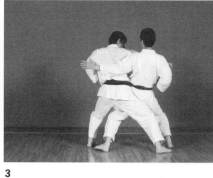

3

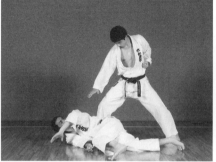

4

5

6

7

Jiyū Kumite No. 13

1. Opponent A (left) and opponent B face off in free-sparring stance.

2–3. A delivers *jōdan kizami-zuki* (photo 2) and then immediately steps behind B while reaching across his chest (photo 3).

4–6. A throws B backward to the floor (photo 4), turns (photo 5), and finishes off with *gyaku-zuki* (photo 6).

7. A recovers and stands upright.

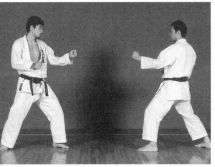

1

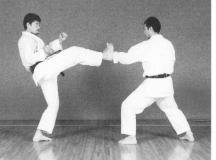

2

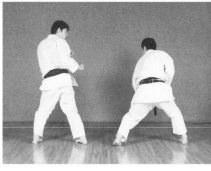

3

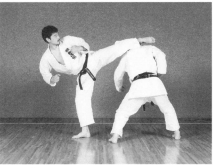

4

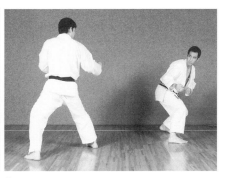

5

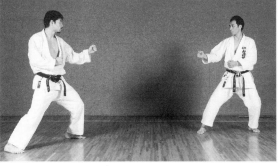

6

Jiyū Kumite No. 14

1. Opponent A (left) and opponent B face off in free-sparring stance.

2. A deflects B's front hand with *mikazuki-geri* (crescent kick).

3–4. The moment A's foot touches the floor (photo 3), he continues turning in the same direction and follows up with *ushiro mawashi-geri* (photo 4).

5–6. A recovers (photo 5) and resumes a free-sparring stance (photo 6).

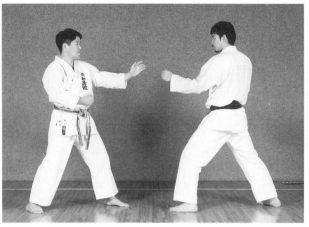

1

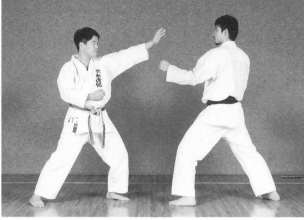

2

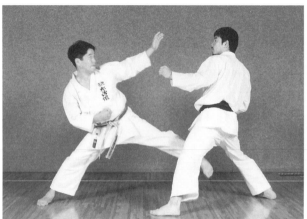

3

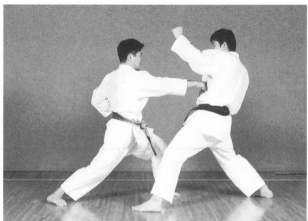

4

Jiyū Kumite No. 15

1. Opponent A (left) and opponent B face off in free-sparring stance.

2–3. A draws B's attention upward (photo 2) and then sweeps B's front leg with *kizami ashi-barai* (leg sweep using the front foot) (photo 3). When executing the leg sweep, keeping the back foot in place makes it difficult for the opponent to anticipate the technique.

4. While B is caught off-balance, A finishes off with *gyaku-zuki*.

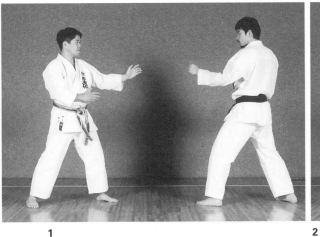

1

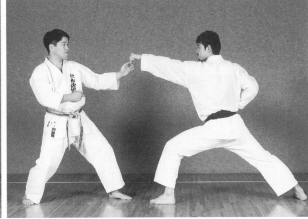

2

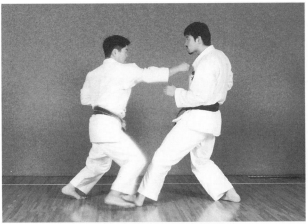

3

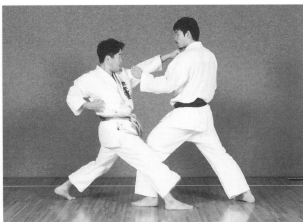

4

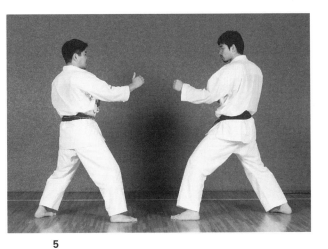

5

Jiyū Kumite No. 16

1. Opponent A (left) and opponent B face off in free-sparring stance.

2–4. A leans away from B's *jōdan kizami-zuki* (photo 2) and then immediately lunges forward, checking B with *jōdan-zuki* (photo 3), and finishing off with *jōdan gyaku-zuki* (photo 4).

5. A recovers and resumes a free-sparring stance.

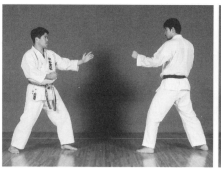 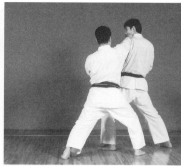

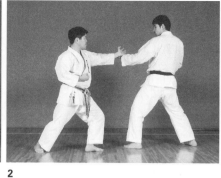

1 2 3

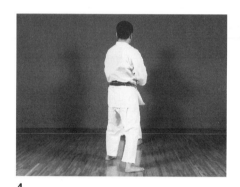 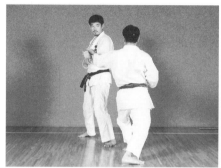 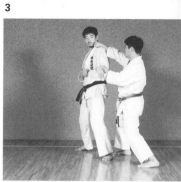

2' 3'

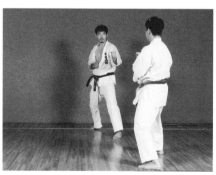

4

Jiyū Kumite No. 17

1. Opponent A (left) and opponent B face off in free-sparring stance.

2–3. A grasps B's front hand (photo 2) and lunges around B to deliver *jōdan mawashi-zuki* (upper-level roundhouse punch) (photo 3).

4. A recovers and resumes a free-sparring stance.

2'–4'. Side-angle views of photos 2 to 4.

4'

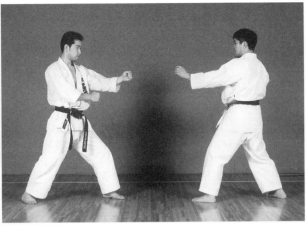

1

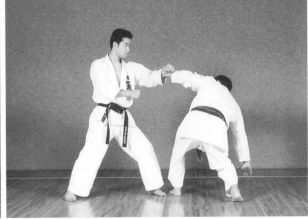

2

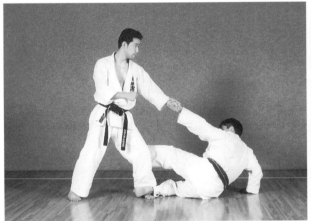

3

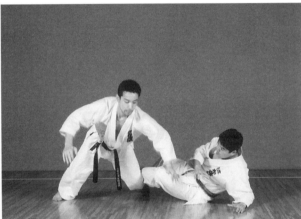

4

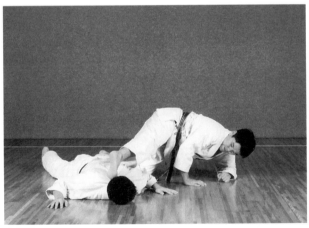

5

Jiyū Kumite No. 18

1. Opponent A (left) and opponent B face off in free-sparring stance.

2. B grasps A's front hand while sliding feet first toward him.

3–4. B catches A's front leg (photo 3) and throws him down with *kani-basami* (crab scissors) (photo 4).

5. B finishes off with *mawashi-geri*.

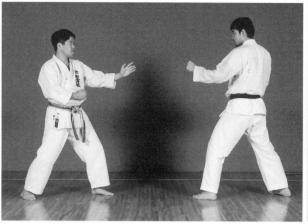

1

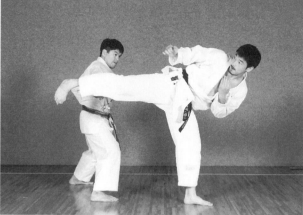

2

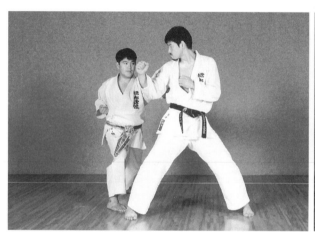

3

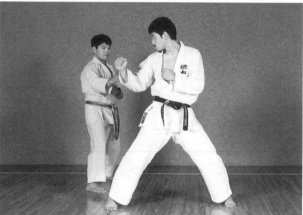

4

Jiyū Kumite No. 19

1. Opponent A (left) and opponent B face off in free-sparring stance.
2. A shifts out of the path of B's *yoko-geri kekomi* (side thrust kick) while blocking with *gedan-barai*.
3. A immediately counters with *chūdan gyaku-zuki*.
4. A recovers and assumes a free-sparring stance.

Jiyū Kumite No. 20 (right page)

1. Opponent A (left) and opponent B face off in free-sparring stance.
2. A shifts to the side, blocking B's *jōdan mawashi-geri* with *haiwan-uke* (back-arm block).
3. A immediately counters with *chūdan gyaku-zuki*.
4. A and B reestablish their *maai* in anticipation of a follow-up exchange.
5. A blocks B's *kizami-zuki* while simultaneously countering with *jōdan kizami mawashi-geri*.
6. A and B recover and assume free-sparring stances.

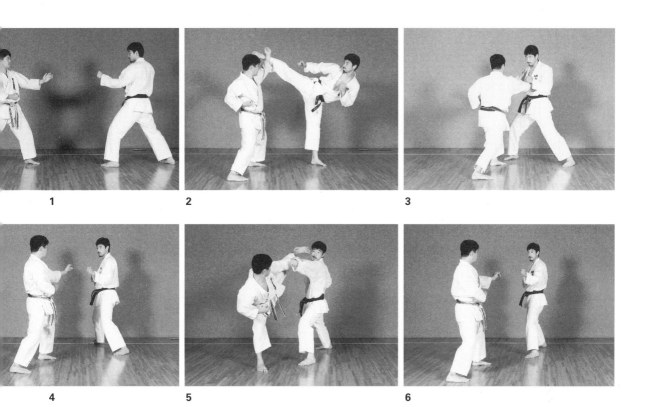

1

2

3

4

5

6

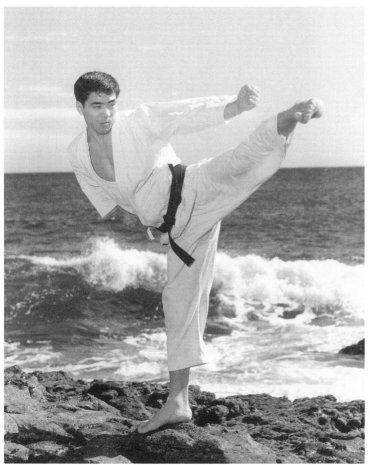

Performing the *kata* Kankū-Dai in Hawaii.

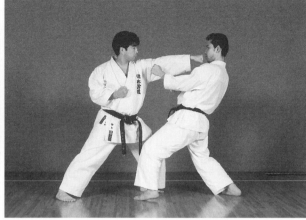

1

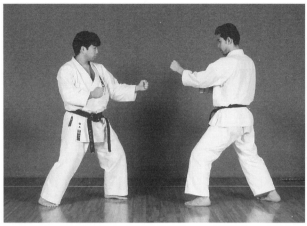

2

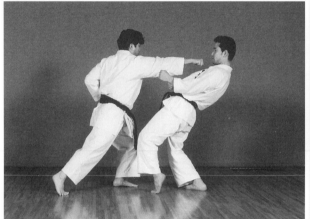

3

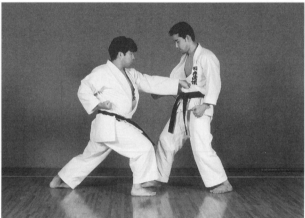

4

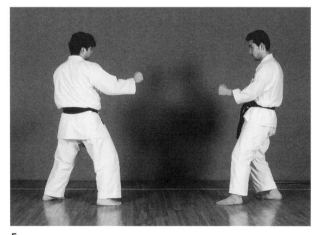

5

Jiyū Kumite No. 21

1. Opponent A (left) and opponent B face off in free-sparring stance.

2. A executes *jōdan kizami-zuki.*

3–4. Lunging forward, A immediately delivers *jōdan gyaku-zuki* (photo 3) followed by *chūdan gyaku-zuki* (photo 4).

5. A recovers and assumes a free-sparring stance.

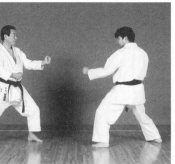

1

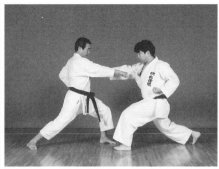

2

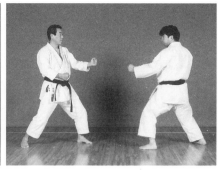

3

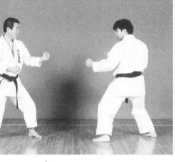

4

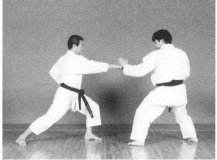

5

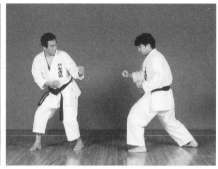

6

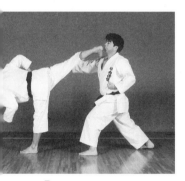

7

Jiyū Kumite No. 22

1. Opponent A (left) and opponent B face off in free-sparring stance.

2. A and B simultaneously attack with *chūdan gyaku-zuki*.

3–4. A and B recover and prepare for a follow-up exchange.

5–7. A checks B with *chūdan gyaku-zuki* (photo 5), draws his front foot back one-half step (photo 6), and then finishes off with *ushiro-geri* (back kick) (photo 7).

HAPPŌ KUMITE (Eight-direction Kumite)

Happō kumite (literally, eight-direction *kumite*) is an applied form of *kumite*. Unlike *tan-ren* (training) *kumite*, *kihon* (basic) *kumite*, *yakusoku* (promise) *kumite*, and *jiyū* (free-style) *kumite*, which involve only a single opponent, *happō kumite* is practiced with multiple opponents, each launching attacks freely from several or all of eight directional points around the defender. The defender must successively shift his body to block each oncoming assault and then execute a counterattack.

If a person were able to defend himself against attacks coming from eight directions, it is unlikely that there would physically be enough room from which an additional attack could be delivered. As such, from a self-defense perspective, if someone were to face more than eight opponents, it would not make much difference if there were ten or there were twenty, as they could only come from approximately eight different directions. This principle represents the thinking behind *happō kumite*.

Regardless of how strong someone may be against a single opponent, if he were not accustomed to facing two or more possible attackers, he would not be able to effectively make use of his strength and techniques in a self-defense capacity. For this reason, we must not forget just how important it is to become adept in such circumstances.

When practicing *happō kumite* it is necessary to combat multiple adversaries over an extended period of time, which requires the coordination of mind and body in such areas as timing, balance, relaxation, concentration, and finesse, as well as agility, endurance, and fluidity of motion for body rotation and body shifting. Accordingly, this form of *kumite* is ideal for developing these abilities. The time allotted is between 30 seconds and two minutes, depending on the level of the defender.

To begin, the defender assumes a free-sparring stance within a circle of a radius equivalent to the distance between the defender's feet when standing in *shizentai* (natural posture). The attackers stand in ready around the defender, maintaining an attacking distance of about two meters (six and a half feet). Although there is no set order for the attacks, each attacker announces the target and technique he will use prior to launching each assault. Following the attack, the attacker immediately returns to the position from which he began. As a rule, only one attacker is allowed to attack at a time. Attacks are launched in succession so as not to provide the defender with an opportunity to rest, with each new attack beginning as soon as it has been confirmed that the defender has decisively countered the previous one.

The defender should make every effort to keep one foot inside of the aforementioned circle, being careful not to let his opponents drive him "into a corner."

The defender must achieve a state of mental preparedness, concentrating the focus in the lower abdomen and awakening every nerve throughout his body to ensure total alertness. At the same time, however, he must remain composed in a relaxed stance while awaiting each attack. With each attack, the defender must accurately assess his opponent's direction, distance, and technique, and react with appropriate body rotation or body shifting while simultaneously blocking, and then follow through with a counterattack. Alternatively, the defender may choose to simultaneously counter while rotating or shifting his body in response to the oncoming attack. The defender must then immediately assume a *shizentai* ready position in preparation for the next assault.

When practicing *happō kumite*, special care must be paid to ensure that breathing does not become erratic. Breathing is an important factor that greatly influences both physical endurance and self-confidence.

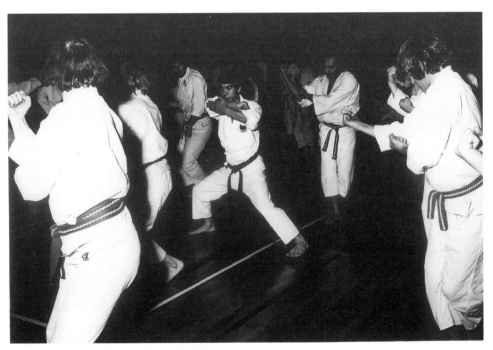

Teaching the *kata* Heian Go-dan in England in 1965.

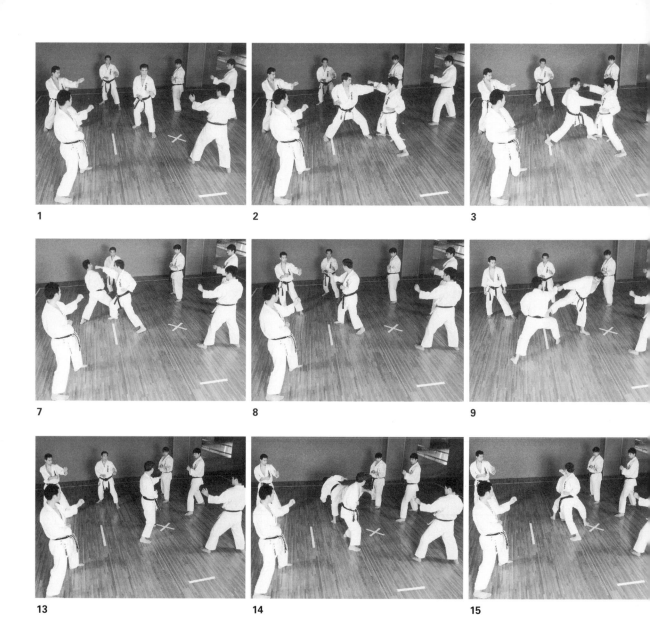

1. The defender (center) assumes a ready position.

2. Defender blocks *jōdan-zuki* (upper-level punch) attack with *tate-shutō uke* (vertical knife-hand block).

3. Defender counters with *chūdan gyaku-zuki* (middle-level reverse punch).

4. Defender recovers and resumes free-sparring stance.

5. Defender blocks *mae-geri* (front snap kick) attack with *gedan-barai* (downward block).

6. Defender pulls back blocking hand.

7. Defender, using the same hand, counters with *jōdan-zuki*.

8. Defender recovers and resumes free-sparring stance.

9. Defender blocks *chūdan-zuki* attack while simultaneously countering with *chūdan mawashi-geri* (middle-level roundhouse kick).

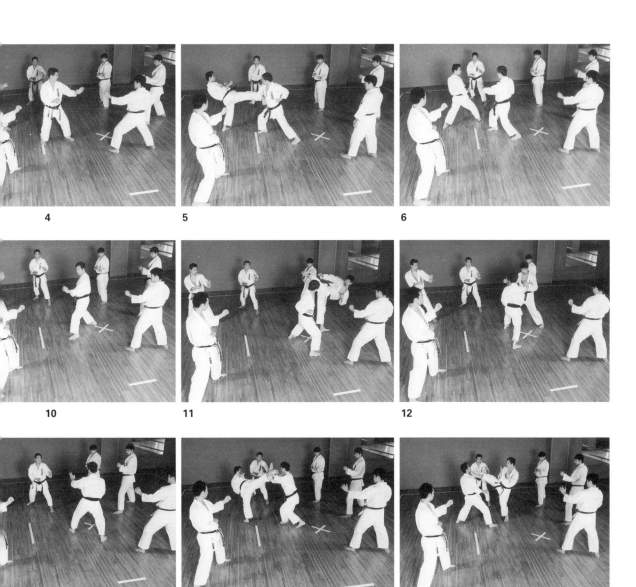

4	5	6
10	11	12
16	17	18

10. Defender recovers and resumes free-sparring stance.

11. Defender blocks *jōdan mawashi-geri* attack with *haiwan-uke* (back-arm block).

12. Defender counters with *chūdan gyaku-zuki*.

13. Defender recovers and resumes free-sparring stance.

14. Defender blocks *ushiro-geri* (back kick) attack with *haiwan-uke*.

15. Defender counters with *jōdan oi-zuki* (upper-level lunge punch).

16. Defender recovers and resumes free-sparring stance.

17. Defender blocks *jōdan mawashi-geri* attack with *tate heikō-uke* (vertical parallel knife-hand block).

18. Defender counters with *mawash-geri*.

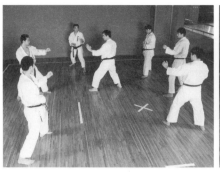

19

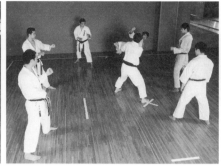

20

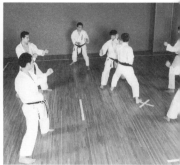

21

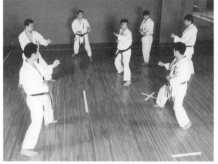

25

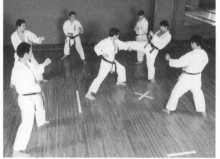

26

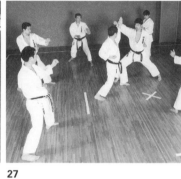

27

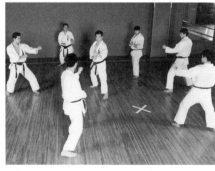

31

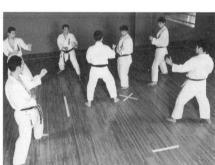

32

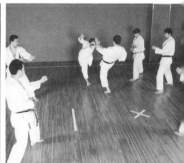

33

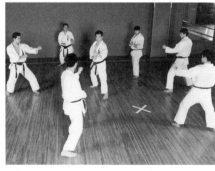

37

19. Defender recovers and resumes free-sparring stance.

20. Defender blocks *yoko-kekomi* (side thrust kick) attack with *gedan-barai*.

21. Defender counters with *uraken-uchi* (back-fist strike).

22. Defender recovers and resumes free-sparring stance.

23. Defender blocks *mae-geri* attack with *gedan jūji-uke* (lower-level X-block).

24. Defender counters with *shutō-uchi* (knife-hand strike).

25. Defender recovers.

26. Defender blocks *mae-geri* attack with *gedan-barai*.

27. Defender blocks subsequent *jōdan jun-zuki* (upper-level front punch) attack with *haiwan-uke*.

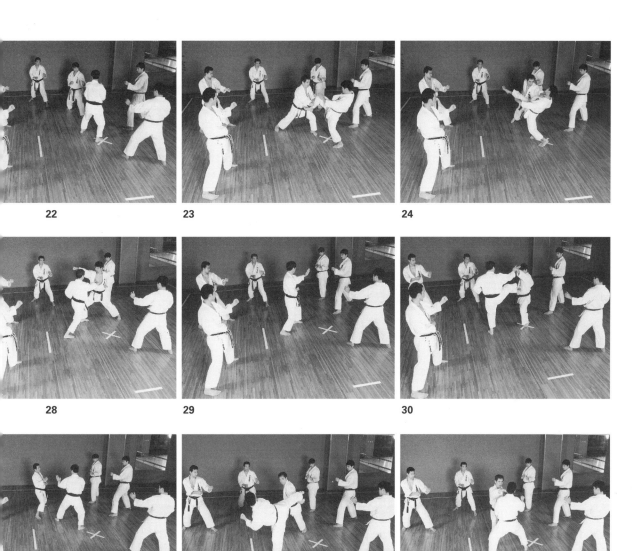

22	23	24
28	29	30
34	35	36

28. Defender counters with *chūdan gyaku-zuki*.

29. Defender recovers and resumes free-sparring stance.

30. Defender blocks *jōdan oi-zuki* attack with *haiwan-uke* while simultaneously countering with *uchi mawashi-geri* (inside roundhouse kick).

31. Defender follows through with *jōdan gyaku-zuki*.

32. Defender recovers and resumes free-sparring stance.

33. Defender blocks *mawashi-geri* attack with *haiwan-uke* while simultaneously countering with *mae-geri*.

34. Defender recovers and resumes free-sparring stance.

35. Defender blocks *ushiro-geri* attack with *gyaku kake-uke* (reverse hooking block).

36. Defender counters with *jōdan jun-zuki*.

37. Defender recovers and resumes free-sparring stance.

TARGET TRAINING

Target training is a special form of training aimed at improving the accuracy of punches, kicks, and strikes, and increasing the efficacy of *kime* (focus) when performing these techniques. As such, it is of particular importance to karate practitioners that participate in non-contact (*sun-dome*) competition.

Lately, when watching *kumite* matches at tournaments, I cannot help but notice how often strong offensive techniques unnecessarily end in failure due to a variety of reasons: the distance (*maai*) between contestants is inappropriate, attacks too frequently miss their intended target, focus is weak, or contact is made. In all likelihood, the true success rate for offensive techniques in karate could be less than that for hits in baseball.

Competitive *kumite* evolved from karate as an art of self-defense. Accordingly, only when punches, kicks, and strikes possess tremendous destructive force, can be delivered at will with absolute precision, and are brought to an immediate halt the instant before they make contact with the intended target, can such *kumite* truly be regarded as karate.

While a *makiwara* (punching board) or sandbag can be used to develop stronger punches, kicks, and strikes, taking full advantage of such powerful techniques becomes unexpectedly difficult when confronting a moving opponent. Therefore it is necessary to practice observing opponents carefully and delivering successive offensive techniques with absolutely no unnecessary motion, ensuring that each attack attains peak explosive power the instant before reaching its target. Target training was created to fulfill this objective.

Although a belt is used in the following examples, a more effective substitute would be a bicycle inner tube filled with beans or rice as it offers a more authentic reaction and feel upon impact. As a general rule, each punch, kick, and strike should "penetrate" the target, traveling beyond the belt or inner tube by a distance of 10 centimeters (about four inches). The reason for this is twofold.

Firstly, in the case of non-contact competition, there is a risk that reflexes and motor functions will grow accustomed to halting techniques just before making contact with the target, which could interfere with the ability to deliver a blow to an opponent's body during an actual encounter. Unless one's skills in competition are equivalent to abilities in actual combat, they cannot be considered karate.

Secondly, only through practicing actually striking a target with one's fists and acquiring the feel of what it is to make contact does it become possible to fully appreciate the importance of controlling attacks. Only then, in my opinion, does it become possible to employ such control. The ability to stop a fist or a foot delivering an attack of lethal force just before it makes contact represents the true meaning of control.

I studied Tai Chi Chuan under Master Yang Ming-Shi (Yō Meiji) and was granted certification as an instructor. I decided to learn the Chinese martial art because it differs greatly from karate and I believed that it would provide me with insight into my karate and enable me to further refine my skills. Indeed, the results proved very beneficial. Studying Tai Chi Chuan helped me develop complementary reflexes, motor functions, and sensory skills.

Depending on the target training exercise, the partner holding the belt or inner tube will either move it back about 35 centimeters (13–14 inches) immediately after the first attack (as in exercise nos. 1, 2, and 5), or hold it in place throughout (as in exercise nos. 3,4 and 6).

The attacker's punches, kicks, and strikes must be driven through the target about 10 centimeters (four inches), executed with speed and force sufficient to make the belt or inner tube emit a "whizzing" sound and whirl around. After delivering the first technique the attacker must immediately confirm the location of the target while simultaneously following through with the second technique.

When performing successive attacks, the abdomen controls the moving of one's center of gravity and the maintaining of balance. The abdomen (*tanden* in Japanese) plays a central role in realizing the comprehensive control required in karate while the hips contribute a supporting function and increase effectiveness. Movement of the hips always involves the abdomen's power, and we must not forget that the strength of the abdomen also conveys energy and vigor.

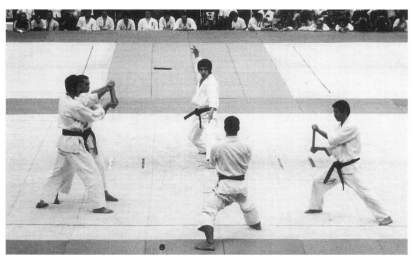

The author performs a demonstration at the second IAKF karate championship tournament, held in 1977 at the Budōkan in Tokyo.

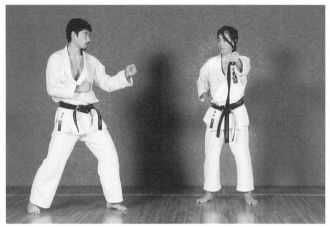

1

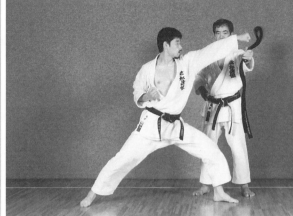

2

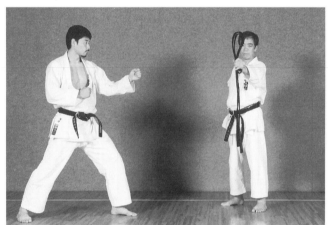

1

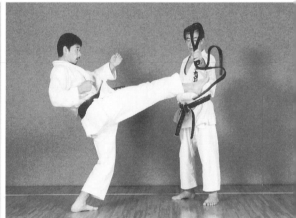

2

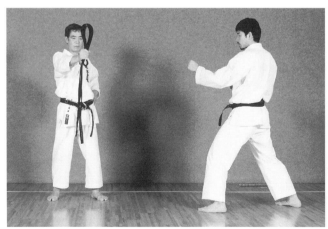

1

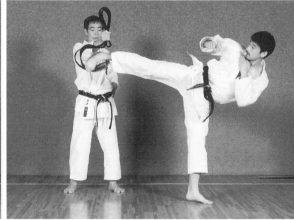

2

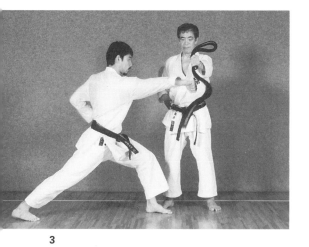

3

Target Training—Basic Movement

1. Ready position.
2. *Jōdan kizami-zuki* (upper-level jab).
3. *Chūdan gyaku-zuki* (middle-level reverse punch).

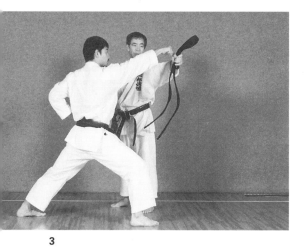

3

Target Training No. 1

1. Ready position.
2. *Chūdan mae-geri* (middle-level front snap kick).
   When executing the kick, it is important to maintain the left-hand-forward upper-body orientation in preparation for the punch that follows.
3. *Jōdan oi-zuki* (upper-level lunge punch).

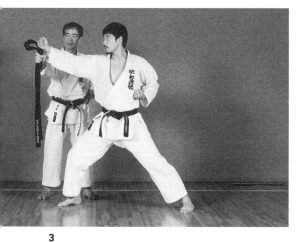

3

Target Training No. 2

1. Ready position.
2. *Chūdan yoko-kekomi* (middle-level side thrust kick).
3. *Jōdan uraken-uchi* (upper-level back-fist strike).

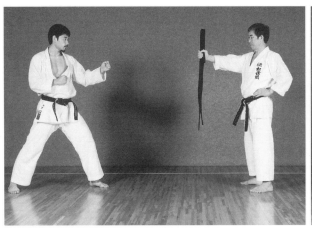

1

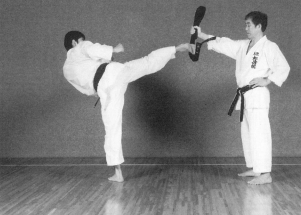

2a

Target Training No. 3

1. Ready position.

2a–2b. *Chūdan mawashi-geri* (middle-level roundhouse kick) (photo 2a) or *jōdan mawashi-geri* (photo 2b).

3. *Jōdan hirate-barai.* (upper-level open-hand sweeping block).

4. *Chūdan gyaku-zuki.*
The punch is delivered at the instant that the kicking foot touches the floor.

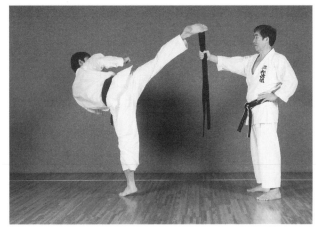

2b

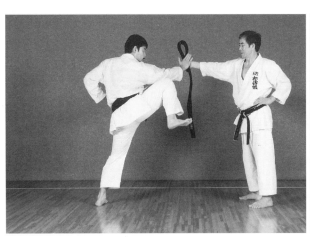

3

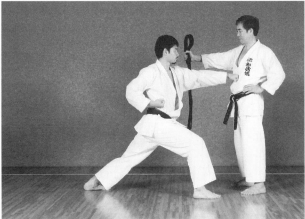

4

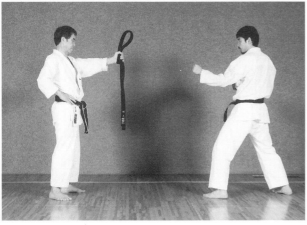

1

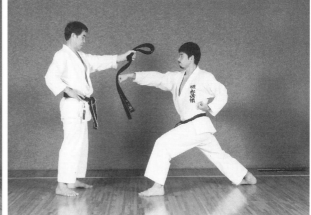

2

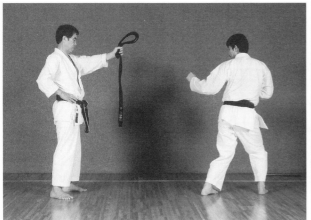

3

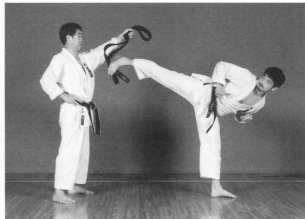

4

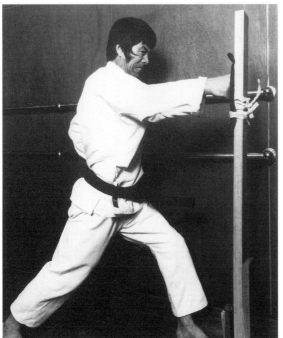

Practicing a reverse punch using a *makiwara*.

Target Training No. 4

1. Ready position.
2. *Chūdan gyaku-zuki.*
3. The punching hand is pulled back at the same time the front foot is drawn back one-half step.
4. *Ushiro-geri* (back kick).

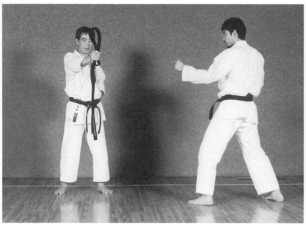

1

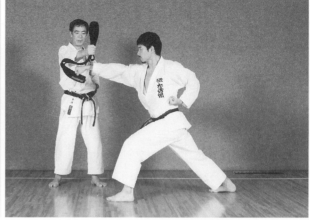

2

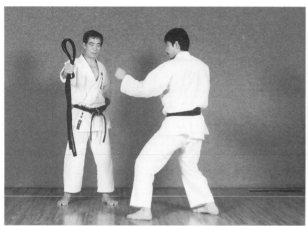

3

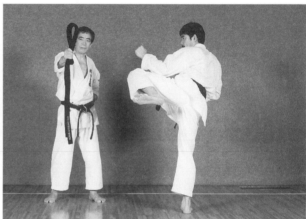

4

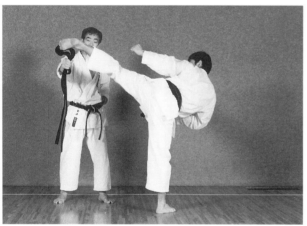

5

Target Training No. 5

1. Ready position.

2. *Chūdan gyaku-zuki.*

3. The punching hand is pulled back at the same time the back foot is drawn forward one-half step.

4. The front foot is raised in preparation to deliver *mawashi-geri.*

5. *Jōdan* (or *chūdan*) *kizami mawashi-geri* (short roundhouse kick).

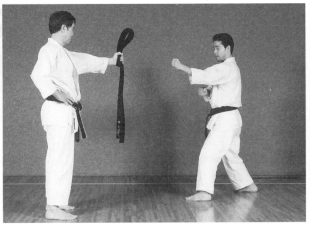

1

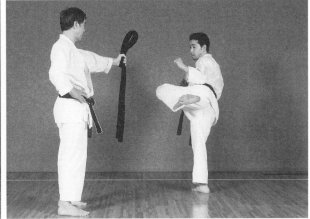

2

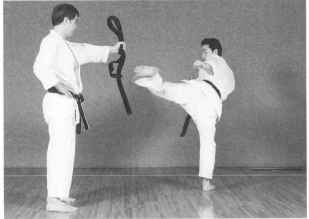

3

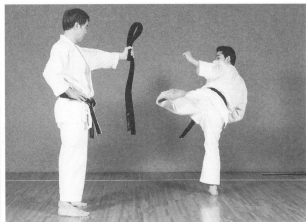

4

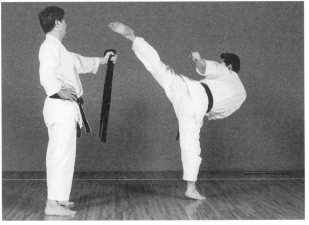

5

Target Training No. 6

1. Ready position.

2. The front foot is raised in preparation to deliver *mawashi-geri*.

3. *Chūdan kizami mawashi-geri.*

4. The kicking foot is retracted, but not placed on the floor.

5. *Jōdan kizami mawashi-geri.*

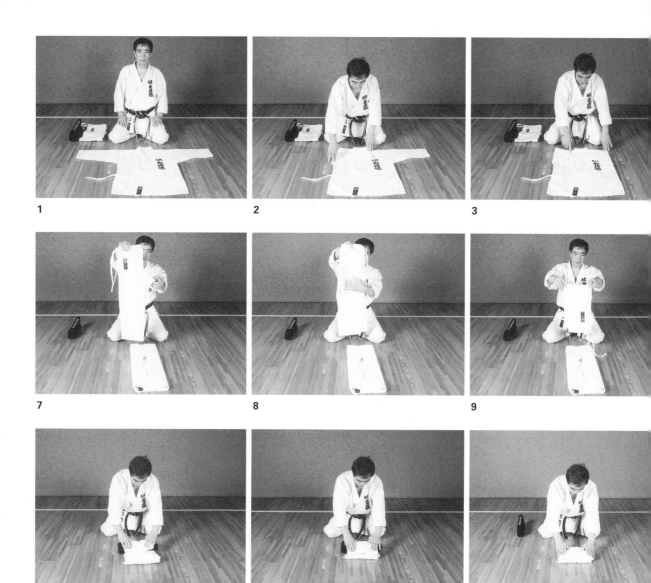

1

2

3

7

8

9

13

14

15

FOLDING A DŌ-GI

1. Place the jacket flat on the floor with the sleeves spread out to each side.

2–3. Fold the sleeves, one at a time, inward across the chest of the jacket at the shoulder seam.

4–5. Fold the outer edges, one at a time, inward towards the center so that the width of the folded jacket is approximately the same as that for the pants once the pants have been folded lengthwise.

6–7. Fold the pants lengthwise so that the name remains on the outside. Fold the triangular flap at the crotch of the pants back toward the side opposite of where the name appears.

8–9. Fold the pants in half so that the name remains on the outside.

10. Place the pants on top of the jacket with the folded edge of the pants aligned above the collar of the jacket.

11. Fold the hem of the jacket back and over the waist of the pants.

12. Place the folded belt on top of the folded jacket and pants.

13–15. Fold the jacket and pants in thirds over the belt, first from the collar, and then from the opposite side.

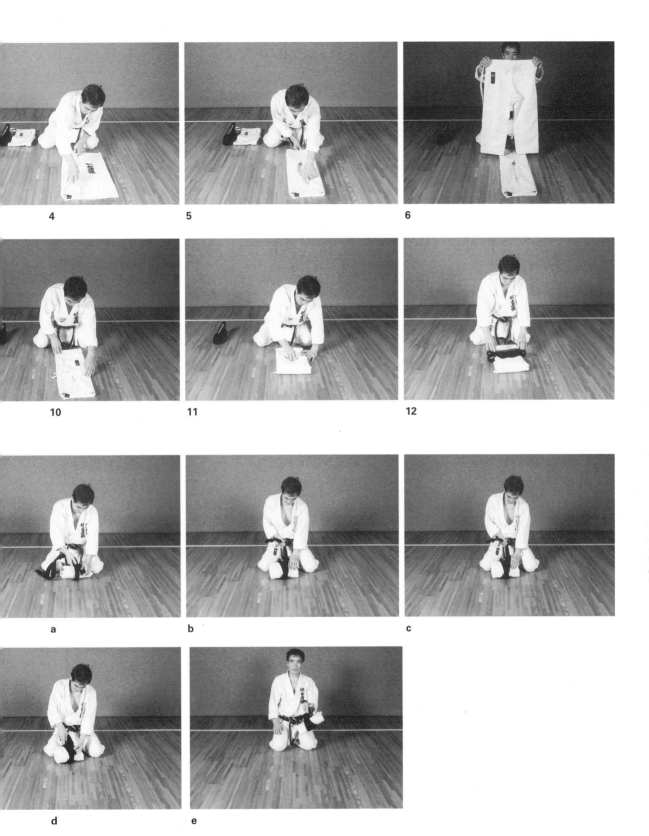

Variation using the belt for carrying

a–c. Fold the jacket and pants as described in steps 1–15 without the belt. Wrap the belt, folded in half, around the jacket and pants.

d–e. Thread the ends of the belt through the loop formed by the folded portion of the belt.

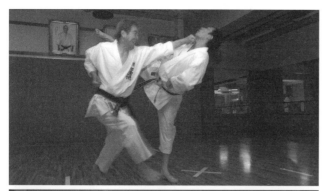

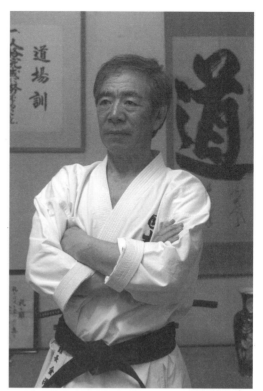

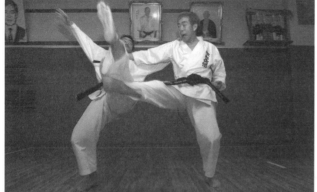

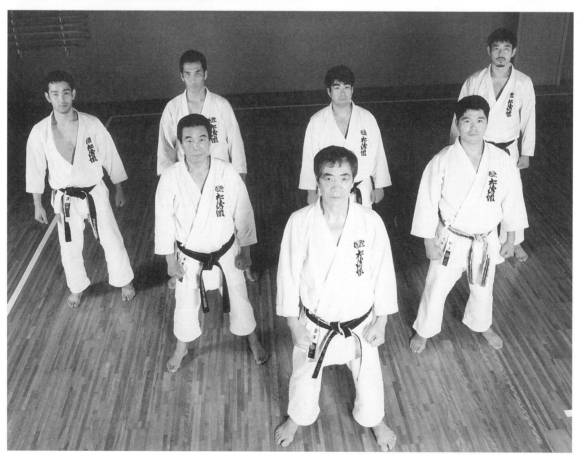

Front: Hirokazu Kanazawa   Second row: (left to right) Shigeyuki Ichihara, Manabu Murakami
Back row: (left to right) Fumitoshi Kanazawa, Shinji Tanaka, Ryūshō Suzuki, Nobuaki Kanazawa

GLOSSARY OF JAPANESE KARATE TERMS

General

Budō: The martial arts

Chūdan: Middle level of the body (chest area)

De-ai: Encounter

Dō-gi: Karate uniform (also *karate-gi*)

Dōjō: Training hall

Empi: Elbow (also *hiji*)

Empi-uchi: Elbow strike

Gedan: Lower level of the body

Gohon kumite: Five-step *kumite*

Gyaku: Reverse or opposite

Haitō: Ridge-hand strike

Hanmi: Half-front-facing position (hips at a 45-degree angle to the front)

Hidari: Left

Hiji: Elbow (also *empi*)

Hiki-te: Pulling hand

Hirate: Open hand

Ippon kumite: One-step *kumite* (either *kihon, kaeshi, jiyū*, or *okuri-jiyū ippon-kumite*)

Jiyū ippon-kumite: Free-style one-step *kumite*

Jiyū kumite: Free sparring

Jōdan: Upper level of the body (face area)

Haishu: Backhand

Happō kumite: Literally eight-direction *kumite*, multi-partner *kumite*

Hiji: Elbow

Hiki-ashi: Pulling foot

Kaeshi ippon-kumite: Attack and counter one-step kumite

Karate-dō: Way or path of karate

Karate-gi: Karate uniform (also *dō-gi*)

Kata: Pre-arranged forms comprising a series of offensive and defensive techniques that are performed individually against an imaginary opponent

Keri: Kick (pronounced "*geri*" when attached to another word, as in *mae-geri*)

Kiai: Loud vocalization timed to coincide with a decisive technique, spirit

Kihon: Basic, the basics

Kihon ippon-kumite: Basic one-step *kumite*

Kihon kumite: Basic *kumite*

Kime: Focus

Kiso kumite: Fundamental *kumite*

Kizami: Refers to a technique performed using the hand or foot positioned in front

Kumite: Sparring

Kyōgi-kumite: Tournament *kumite*

Maai: Distance maintained between opponents during *kumite*

Mae: Front

Makiwara: Punching board

Migi: Right

Nukite: Spear hand

Okuri jiyū-ippon-kumite: Follow-through free-style one-step *kumite*

Oss: Verbal greeting exchanged between karate practitioners (see "Lessons From the Master," pp. 12–19)

Rei: Bow, bowing (see "Rei," pp. 22–23)

Reigi: Manners

Sahō: Etiquette (see "Rei," pp. 22–23)

Sanbon kumite: Three-step *kumite*

Setsu: Principles (see "Rei and Setsu," p. 26)

Shiai kumite: Match-style *kumite*

Shihon-nukite: Four-finger spear hand

Shutō: Knife-hand

Sokumen: Side

Sonoba-zuki: Punching while standing in place

Sun-dome: Bringing attacks to a sudden halt just before making contact with the target (one *sun* is approx. 3 cm., or 1 1/4 inches)

Tachi: Stance (pronounced "*dachi*" when attached to another word, as in *zenkutsu-dachi*)

Tai-sabaki: Body shifting

Tanden: Abdomen

Tanren-kumite: Training *kumite*

Teishō: Palm-heel

Tenshin: Body rotation

Tsuki: Punch (pronounced "*zuki*" when attached to another word, as in *gyaku-zuki*)

Tsuki-te: Punching hand

Uchi: Strike

Uchi-te: Striking hand

Uke: Block

Ushiro: Back

Yakusoku-kumite: Promise sparring

Yoko: Side

Zanshin: A state of physical and mental preparedness following an attack

Zenmi: Full-front-facing position (hips facing the front)

Stances

Fudō-dachi: Rooted stance

Hachiji-dachi: Open V stance (also *hachiji-dachi shizentai*)

Hanmi: Half-front-facing position (hips at a 45-degree angle to the front)

Hiza kakushi-dachi: Hidden-knee stance

Kiba-dachi: Straddle-leg stance

Kōkutsu-dachi: Back stance

Musubi-dachi: Closed V stance

Neko ashi-dachi: Cat stance

Shizentai: Natural posture

Tachi: Stance (pronounced "*dachi*" when attached to another word, as in *zenkutsu-dachi*)

Uke-te: Blocking hand

Zenkutsu-dachi: Front stance

Zenmi: Full-front-facing position (hips facing the front)

Hand/Arm Techniques

Age-uke: Rising block

Awase seiryūtō-uke: Two-handed ox-jaw block

Choku-zuki: Straight punch

Chūdan gyaku ura-zuki: Middle-level reverse close punch

Chūdan gyaku-zuki: Middle-level reverse punch

Chūdan hiji-uke: Middle-level elbow block

Chūdan haiwan-uke: Middle-level back-arm block

Chūdan jun-zuki: Middle-level front punch

Chūdan kizami-zuki: Middle-level jab

Chūdan mawashi-uke: Middle-level round block, middle-level hooking block

Chūdan oi-zuki: Middle-level lunge punch

Chūdan shutō-uke: Middle-level knife-hand block

Chūdan soto ude-uke: Middle-level outside-to-inside block

Chūdan tate shihon-nukite: Middle-level vertical four-finger spear hand

Chūdan teishō-uchi: Middle-level palm-heel strike

Chūdan teishō-uke: Middle-level palm-heel block

Chūdan uchi ude-uke: Middle-level inside-to-outside block

Chūdan ura gyaku-zuki: Middle-level close reverse punch

Chūdan yoko empi-uchi: Middle-level side elbow strike

Empi-uchi: Elbow strike

Gedan-barai: Downward block

Gedan gyaku osae-uke: Lower-level reverse pressing block

Gedan jūji-uke: Lower-level X-block

Gedan seiryūtō-uke: Lower-level ox-jaw block

Gedan-uke: Downward block

Gyaku age-uke: Reverse rising block

Gyaku chūdan shutō-uke: Reverse middle-level knife-hand block

Gyaku gedan-barai: Reverse downward block

Gyaku gedan-uke: Reverse downward block

Gyaku kake-uke: Reverse hooking block

Gyaku oi-zuki: Reverse lunge punch

Gyaku osae-uke: Reverse pressing block

Gyaku sukui-uke: Reverse scooping block

Gyaku ura-zuki: Reverse close punch

Gyaku-zuki: Reverse punch

Haishu juji-uke: Backhand X-block

Haitō-uchi: Ridge-hand strike

Haiwan nagashi-uke: Back-arm sweeping block

Haiwan-uke: Back-arm block

Harai-uke: Sweeping block

Heikō-uke: Parallel block (also *tate heikō shutō-uke* or *tate heikō-uke*)

Hiji-uke: Elbow block

Hiki-te: Pulling hand

Hirate-barai: Open-hand sweeping block

Hirate-uke: Open-hand block

Jōdan age-uke: Upper-level rising block

Jōdan gyaku-zuki: Upper-level reverse punch

Jōdan haishu juji-uke: Upper-level backhand X-block

Jōdan haitō-uchi: Upper-level ridge-hand strike

Jōdan haiwan-uke: Upper-level back-arm block

Jōdan harai-uke: Upper-level sweeping block

Jōdan heikō-uke: Upper-level parallel block

Jōdan hirate-barai: Upper-level open-hand sweeping block

Jōdan jun-zuki: Upper-level front punch

Jōdan kizami-zuki: Upper-level jab

Jōdan mawashi-zuki: Upper-level roundhouse punch

Jōdan nagashi-uke: Upper-level sweeping block

Jōdan oi-zuki: Upper-level lunge punch

Jōdan shutō jūji-uchi: Upper-level knife-hand X-strike

Jōdan shutō-uchi: Upper-level knife-hand strike

Jōdan tate shutō-uke: Upper-level vertical knife-hand block

Jōdan tate teishō-uchi: Upper-level upward palm-heel strike

Jōdan uraken-uchi: Upper-level back-fist strike

Jōdan ushiro mawashi empi-uchi: Upper-level back roundhouse elbow strike

Jōdan yama-uke: Upper-level mountain block

Jōdan yoko uraken-uchi: Upper-level side back-fist strike

Jōdan-zuki: Upper-level punch

Jūji-uchi: X-strike

Jūji-uke: X-block

Jun-zuki: Front punch

Kake-uke: Hooking block

Kizami-zuki: Jab

Mae empi-uchi: Forward elbow strike

Mawashi empi-uchi: Roundhouse elbow strike

Mawashi-uke: Round block, hooking block

Mawashi-zuki: Roundhouse punch

Morote uchi ude-uke: Augmented inside-to-outside block

Nagashi-uke: Sweeping block

Nukite: Spear hand

Oi-zuki: Lunge punch

Osae-uke: Pressing block

Seiryūtō-uke: Ox-jaw block

Shihon-nukite: Four-finger spear hand

Shutō: Knife-hand

Shutō jūji-uchi: Knife-hand X-strike

Shutō-uchi: Knife-hand strike

Shutō-uke: Knife-hand block

Sokumen jōdan uke: Side upper-level block

Sonoba-zuki: Punching while standing in place

Soto ude-uke: Outside-to-inside block

Sukui-uke: Scooping block

Tate enmpi-uchi: Upward elbow strike

Tate heikō shutō-uke: Vertical parallel knife-hand block (also *tate heikō-uke* or *heikō-uke*)

Tate heikō-uke: Vertical parallel knife-hand block (also *tate heikō shutō-uke* or *heikō-uke*)

Tate-ken: Vertical fist

Tate-zuki: Vertical-fist punch

Tate shihon-nukite: Vertical four-finger spear hand

Tate shutō: Vertical knife-hand

Tate shutō-uke: Vertical knife-hand block

Tate teishō-uchi: Upward palm-heel strike

Teishō-uchi: Palm-heel strike

Teishō-uke: Palm-heel block

Tsuki: Punch (pronounced *"zuki"* when attached to another word, as in *gyaku-zuki*)

Tsuki-te: Punching hand

Uchi: Strike

Uchi-te: Striking hand

Uchi ude-uke: Inside-to-outside block

Uke: Block

Uke-te: Blocking hand

Uraken-uchi: Back-fist strike

Ura gyaku-zuki: Close reverse punch

Ura-zuki: Close punch

Ushiro chūdan-barai: Back middle-level block

Ushiro mawashi empi-uchi: Back roundhouse elbow strike

Ushiro shutō-uchi: Back knife-hand strike

Yama-uke: Mountain block

Yoko empi-uchi: Side elbow strike

Yoko uraken-uchi: Side back-fist strike

Leg Techniques

Ashi-barai: Leg sweep

Chūdan kizami-geri: Middle-level short front kick

Chūdan kizami mawashi-geri: Middle-level short roundhouse kick

Chūdan mae-geri: Middle-level front snap kick

Chūdan mawashi-geri: Middle-level roundhouse kick

Chūdan yoko-kekomi: Middle-level side thrust kick

De-ai chūdan mae-geri: Encounter middle-level front snap kick

Gedan kizami mawashi-geri: Lower-level short roundhouse kick

Jōdan kekomi: Upper-level thrust kick

Jōdan kizami mawashi-geri: Upper-level short roundhouse kick

Jōdan mawashi-geri: Upper-level roundhouse kick

Jōdan ushiro mawashi-geri: Upper-level back roundhouse kick

Jōdan ushiro uchi mawashi-geri: Upper-level back inside roundhouse kick

Kani-basami: Crab scissors

Kekomi: Thrust kick

Kizami ashi-barai: Leg sweep using the front foot

Kizami-geri: Short kick (kick using the front leg)

Kizami mawashi-geri: Short roundhouse kick

Kizami ushiro mawashi-geri: Short back roundhouse kick

Kizami yoko-geri: Short side kick

Keri: Kick (pronounced *"geri"* when attached to another word, as in *mae-geri*)

Kizami ashi-barai: Short leg sweep

Mae-geri: Front snap kick

Mawashi-geri: Roundhouse kick

Mikazuki-geri: Crescent kick

Nami-ashi: Inward foot snap

Suri-ashi: A "gliding" step, without raising the foot

Tobi-geri: Jump kick

Uchi mawashi-geri: Inside roundhouse kick

Ushiro-geri: Back kick

Ushiro mawashi-geri: Back roundhouse kick

Ushiro uchi mawashi-geri: Back inside roundhouse kick

Yoko-geri: Side kick

Yoko-geri ke-age: Side snap kick

Yoko-geri kekomi: Side thrust kick (also *yoko-kekomi*)

Yoko-kekomi: Side thrust kick (also *yoko-geri kekomi*)

SKIF CONTACT LIST

Algeria
Rguiba Boumedine
10 Rue Francois, Jarsaillon,
Victor Hugo, Oran 31000
PHONE: (213) 6 467504

Argentina
Coronel Mario Oscar
Asociacion Argentina S.K.I.
9 de Julio 4179-Mar del Plata-
Provincia de Buenos Aires
PHONE: (54) 223 473 6709
FAX: (54) 223 474 9031
E-MAIL: argentina_ski@hotmail.com

Australia
Brian Cox
SKI Australia, Memberships Officer
61 Barnes Crescent, Menai,
NSW 2234
PHONE/FAX: (61) 02 9543 6028
E-MAIL: briancox@primus.com.au

John Brailey
32 Wordsworth Avenue,
Bateau Bay, NSW 2261
PHONE: (61) 02 4334 4999
FAX: (61) 0243 237040 /
(61) 0243 231100

Lex Mckinley
SKI Australia, President
35 Short Street, Joondanna,
Perth WA6060
PHONE/FAX: (61) 08 9444 3434

Tim Stephenson
SKI Australia, Secretary
102 9th Avenue, Maylands,
WA6051
PHONE: (61) 08 9271 6808
FAX: (61) 08 9221 7701

Zivko Delevski
SKI Australia, Coaching Coordinator
15 Stewart Avenue,
Matraville, NSW 2036
PHONE/FAX: (61) 02 9661 6286

Robert Mansberg, Dr.
SKI Australia, Treasurer
4/7B Judge Street, Randwick,
NSW 2031
c/o Maroubra Seals 212
Marine Parade,
Maroubra Beach, NSW 2035
PHONE: (61) 02 9439 2299
FAX: (61) 02 9349 5658
PHONE: (61) 02 9398 5304
E-MAIL: mansberg@nucmed.rpa.cs.
nsw.gov.au

Austria
Erich Laufer
SKI Austria, President
St. Peter Hauptstr. 33d,
A-8042 Graz
PHONE: (43) 699-1110-8912

Norio Kawasoe
SKI Austria, Chief Instructor
Ebenhochgasse 14a,
A-6840 Gotzis
PHONE: (43) 5523 64781

Azerbaijan
Yashar Bashirov
Baku,Y. Vezirov Str.,
123 apt. 33
PHONE: (7) 994 12 906060 /
(7) 994 12 975168 /
(7) 994 12 975031
FAX: (7) 994 12 929288 /
(7) 994 12 931153
E-MAIL: wkf@karate-az.com

Bahamas
Patricia Fergeuson
Academy of Martial Arts
International
No.2 Wongs Plaza Madaira st,
Palmdale Nassau
PHONE/FAX: (242) 356 5460
E-MAIL: ZANSHIN@Batelnet.bs

Bangladesh
Humayun Kabir Jewel
SKI Bangladesh
153/KA, East Raza Bazar
Tejgaon, Dhaka-1215
PHONE: (880) 2 8125932 (OFFICE) /
(880) 2 8110603
FAX: (880) 2 8110603 /
(880) 2 8315369
E-MAIL: kekko@dhaka.net

Padamsee Rani Bilkees
Bengal School of Shotokan
Rd 2, Lane 2, Old D.O.H.S.
Banani, Dhaka
PHONE: (8802) 9895929 /
(8802) 9860631
FAX: (8802) 9882645
E-MAIL: tigress@citechco.net

MD. Moazzem Hossain Sento
55/1 Puranapaltan Lane
(Banglabhaban), Dhaka-1000
PHONE: (880) 02 404312
FAX: (880) 02 408088 /
(880) 02 9557745

Barbados
Joel Linton
P.O. Box 565, Bridgetown,
PHONE: (1) 246 436 4454
FAX: (1) 246 431 0941

Belgium
Luc De Dycker
S.K.I.F Belgium
Via Pergolesi 17 09045
Quartu (CA) Italia
PHONE: (32) 39070821215 /
(32) 075 581955 (MOBILE)
FAX: (32) 39070821215
E-MAIL: skif.belgium@libero.it

Stephane Castrique
Van Duyststraat 37,
B-2100 Deurne
PHONE: (32) 3 326 4107
FAX: (32) 3 326 5722
E-MAIL: stephane.castrique@skibf.be

Benin
Raimi Mansovrou
P/C/ Agossou Frederic,
B.P. 1571 Porto-Novo-229

Brazil
Lodson Espindola
SKI Brazil, International Events
Manager
Rua Galo Branco, 210-Ilha do
Governador-Rio deJaneiro-RJ
CEP : 21941-220
PHONE/FAX: (55) 21 393 6044

Teruo Furusho
Haddock Lobo No. 1-Estacio
CEP 20211-260, Rio de Janeiro
PHONE/FAX: (55) 21 393 6044
E-MAIL: shotokanbrasil@yahoo.
com.br

Burkina Fasso
Traore Ferix Ibrahim
P.O. Box 01, BP 1471,
Ouagadougou 01
PHONE: (225) 307175

Canada
Antonio Terra
SKIF Toronto
114 Dundas Street West,
Toronto, Ontario
PHONE: (1) 416 536 2480

John Gilbert
SKIF Liboire
67 St. Patrice, Li Boire,
Quebec J0H 1R0
PHONE: (1) 450 793 4189

Kenzo Dozono
SKIF Belleville
52 Chatham Street, Belleville,
Ontario K8N 3S4
PHONE: (1) 613 962 8551
FAX: (1) 613 962 1485
E-MAIL: dozono@sympatico.ca

Larry Bowlby
SKIF London
428 Moore Street, London,
Ontario N6C 2C2
PHONE: (1) 519 434 1561

Martin Hunter
SKIF Canmore
130 Coyote Way, Canmore,
Alberta T1W 2A6
PHONE: (1) 403 609 3042

Peter Tanko
SKIF Hamilton
671 Fennel Avenue East,
Hamilton, Ontario L8V 1V3
PHONE: (1) 905 574 9377

Roger Lagace
SKIF Quebec
Academie D'Arts Martiaux
101 Normandin,
St-Alphonse-de-Granby,
Quebec,Joe,2A0
PHONE: (1)-450-372-4741

Chile
Hernan Beltran Silva
Casilla 3826, Conception
PHONE: (56) 41 422865
FAX: (56) 41 215770
E-MAIL: skifchile@hotmail.com

Taizo Takahashi
SKI Chile, General Secretary
Padre Roman 4804,
Vitacura, Santiago
PHONE: (56) 2 228 5350

Cloatia
Brajkovic Davor
SKI Hrvatska
U1. A. Negri 42,
HR-Vrsar 52450
PHONE: (385) 52 441311
FAX: (385) 52 441602

Colombia
Baronio Cifuentes Medina
Union S.K.I. de Colombia
Academia Samurai,
Avenida Boyaca No. 55-41,
Barrio Normandia, Bogota
PHONE: (57) 1 263 1768
E-MAIL: skicolombia@hotmail.com
ski_colombia@latinmail.com
skicolombia@latinmail.com

Comoros
Madi Said
Federation Comorienne de Karate
B.P. 2433, Moroni.
PHONE/FAX: (269) 736122

Costa Rica
Alexander Vargas Rodriguez
Casa Mercedes Sur Heredea,
Frente Mini, Super La Perla
FAX: (506) 261 1022

Cote D'Ivoire
Yao Koffi Julien Ramos
S.K.I.C.I., President
P.O. Box. 25 B.P.2037 Abidjan 25
Nicolas Tanoh
PHONE: (225) 07 57 88 27 /
(225) 07 39 02 78
FAX: (225) 21 27 29 12
E-MAIL: skicii@yahoo.fr

Cuba
Nubia Bregado Gutierrez
Calle 21, No. 1053,
Entre 12 y 14, Vedado, Habana
PHONE: (53) 537 333198, 333215
FAX: (53) 537 333088

Denmark
Bruno Jensen
SKI Denmark, Chief Instructor
Elme Alle 20,
2610 Hvidovre
PHONE: (45) 31 782344

Jan Spatzek
SKI-Denmark (HEAD OFFICE)
Kastanievej 20, 7470 Karup J.
PHONE: (45) 97 102482
FAX: (45) 97 100330
E-MAIL: skif@skif.dk /
shotokan@skif.dk

Viggo Johannsen
Bragesvej 15, DK-8230,
Aabyhoej
PHONE/FAX: (45) 86 156309
E-MAIL: hagen.johannsen@mail.sto-
fanet.dk

Ecuador
Gilles H. Blain
Ambassador Hotel, Casilla 17-07,
8757 Quito
FAX: (593) 2 503712

Fiji
Parmesh Nand
89 Mead Road Tamavua,
Suva

France
Franco D'Aloia
2 Rue de Archers 80000 Amiens
PHONE: (33) 3 2292 5856
E-MAIL: honbu@nnx.com

Marcel Fabre
14, Av. de L'Europe,
78160 Marley Le Roi
PHONE: (33) 1 39 164679 /
(33) 1 49 076102
FAX: (33) 1 39 164679

Georgia
Zurab Lezhava
Georgian Shotokan Karate-Do
Association
16 Rustaveli Avenue,
380008 Tbilisi
PHONE: (995) 32 293808
FAX: (995) 32 987583 /
(995) 32 232688

Germany
Eugen Landgraf
Adensuer Str. 50, 73433 Aalen
PHONE/FAX: (49) 7361 971799
E-MAIL: landgraf@skid.de

Akio Nagai
SKI Germany, Chief Instructor
Kaiserstrasse 30, 4018 Langenfeld
PHONE: (49) 217 371875 /
(49) 172 8908943 (MOBILE)

Alexander Schifferer
SKI Germany, Secretary
Kirchbergerstrabe 15,
84359 Simbach/Inn
PHONE: (49) 08571 3507

Hajime Tomita
SKI Germany, International Senior
Adviser
LTK REISEBURO, City Center
Immermannstrabe 13,
D-40210, Dusseldorf
PHONE: (49) 211 936930
FAX: (40) 211 351057 /
(49) 221 4060429

Greece
George P. Panayiotides
SKI Greece, President
178, 3rd Septemvriou Street & Ag.
Meletioy 11251, Athens
PHONE: (30) 1 862 2236 /
(30) 683 1875 (HOME) /
(30) 945 895080
FAX: (30) 683 1875

Nikitas Zarouchliotis
SKI Greece, Technical Committee
Hellenic Traditional Karate
Federation

222 El. Venizelou Street,
175 63 P. Faliro, Athens
PHONE: (30) 1 983 2753
FAX: (30) 1 982 2356, 856 2924

Greenland
Eriksen Kim Bohmert
Nuuk Shotokan Karate-Do
PB.749, DK-3900 Nuuk
PHONE: (299) 299 324143
E-MAIL: lissiottosen@yahoo.dk

Guatemala
Manuel Aguilar
15 Avenue, 6-29, Zona 12
PHONE: (502) 712562

Guyana
Anthony Akbar Ignatius Durjan
Guyana Amateur Karate Association
P.O. Box 10213,
G.P.O.-Robb Street, Georgetown
PHONE/FAX: (592) 2 59798

Hong Kong
Ricky Wan
Shotokan Karatedo of Hong Kong
PHONE: (852) 9027 7394

Philip Kwok, Dr.
SKI Yudansha-kai, Chairman
Shotokan Karate of Hong Kong
Wing On Centre7/F.,
211 Des Voeux Road Central
PHONE: (852) 2852 1827
FAX: (852) 2541 2585
E-MAIL: philipkwok@compuserve.
com

William S. Wong
Shotokan Karate of Hong Kong
PHONE: (852) 2852 1879
FAX: (852) 2541 2482, 2850 6077
E-MAIL: contact@shotokan-karate-
hk.com

Hungary
Miklos Toth
SKI Hungary, President
Fo u. 4.
I/1, 1011 Budapest

Totisz Andras
SKI Hungary, International Affairs
PHONE: (36) 1 1409631

Fridrich Gyorgy
SKIF Hungary
Vecses Hunyadi u. 9/A H-2220
PHONE/FAX: (36) 29 351 559

India
Shekhar Chandra
Association of Shotokan
Karate-Do, India
48/2A, Sector-2, Gole Market,
New Delhi 110001
PHONE: (91) 11 374 7260 /
(91) 11 247 6208 /
(98) 11 873828
E-MAIL: chandrasheekhar_ski@
yahoo.co.uk

Devavrta P. Bhatt
A6/8-35, Jeevah Sahtosh Ltc.,
Colony Borivli (West),
Bombay-Hoo 103
PHONE: (91) 22 661731

J. Ghosh
Indian Head Office
4/2, Rammonhan Roy Road,
Calcutta-9
PHONE: (91) 33 35 1358

K. N. S. Pillai
Shotokan Karate Association of
India
P.O. Box 8104,
Bandra (East), Bombay 400-051
PHONE: (91) 22 822 9555

K.V. Subramanyan
Shotokan Karate-Do International
India
605, 7th Main, B.D. A. Houses,
Domlur, Bangalore 560 071
PHONE: (91) 80 5350500
E-MAIL: subramanyanv@hotmail.
com

Satnam Singh Happy
Shotokan Karate-Do Institute
(India)
144 Vishnu Gardens,
Vaha Vishnu, New Delhi 18
PHONE: (91) 11 516 8321
FAX: (91) 11 557 0833

Singh Ram Babu
Friends Club LTD
763 First Floor, Sunlight Colony-
2nd New Delhi 100 014
PHONE: (91) 011 26342302 /
(91) 00 9810191546
E-MAIL: rambabusingh@hotmail.com

T. K. Rajan
B-217, Packet B, DDA Flats,
Sukhdev Vihar,
New Delhi 110025
PHONE/FAX: (91) 11 684 3225

Indonesia
Forki
Federasi Olahrage Karate-Do
Indonesia
Pintul, Stadion Utama Senayan,
Jakarta
PHONE: (62) 021 573 2033 /
(62) 021 573 1632

E. Tando
SKI Indonesia, Chairman
Aldiron Hero Group
Wisma Aldiron Dirgantara,
Suite 200,
Jalan Gatot Subroto Kav. 72,
Jakarta 12780
PHONE: (62) 021 790 2242 /
(62) 081 693 5107 (MOBILE) /
(62) 081 685 2079 (MOBILE, MR.
ASRIL AZHARI)
FAX: (62) 021 799 1786 /
(62) 021 794 9278
E-MAIL: aldironl@aldiron.com /
inkado@ekilat.com

Iran
Manuchher Aslanian
1208 Valiasr Avenue,
Above Park Saee, Teheran
PHONE: (98) 021 888 5291
FAX: (98) 021 524 4553

Ireland
Abe McCarthy
SKI Ireland, Chairman
5 Silverdale Avenue,
Ballinlough, Cork
PHONE: (353) 21 291741
FAX: (353) 21 276484
E-MAIL: mcc@eircom.net

Greg Manning
SKI Ireland, General Secretary
Roseview, 7 Meadowpark Avenue,
Ballyvolane, Cork
PHONE/FAX: (353) 21 508022
E-MAIL: gregmanning@eircom.net

Israel
Avi Klau
Ahad Ha'am 8/A St. 7,
38224 Hadera

PHONE: (972) 06 6322249 /
(972) 06 6344660
FAX: (972) 06 6334776

Danny Hakim
Rashba-Levy, Ohad
SKI Jsrael
Emek st. 1 Kiriat tivon 36084
PHONE: (00972) 4 983 7892 /
(00972) 51 25 94 28 (MOBILE)
FAX: (972) 04 983 7892
E-MAIL: ohadsu@newmail.net

Italy
Toshio Yamada
c/o Sig. Bwonalloggi Giulio
Via Gherardi silvestro 44 Int. 7,
00146 Roma
PHONE/FAX: (39) 06 556 6362

Masaru Miura
Via Sammartini 40,
20125 Milano
PHONE: (39) 02 6669 4269 /
(03) 02 655 2080 (HOME)
FAX: (39) 02 6669 7883

Kazakhstan
Vyacheslav Savckiv
198-4, Mirzoyan St.,
Almaty 480096

Kenya
Kisofero Alirajab Mwadufu
S.K.I.F.-Kenya
P.O. Box 89974,
Mombasa, 80100
PHONE: (254) 733 885942
FAX: (254) 11 230845
E-MAIL: skifkenya@hotmail.com

Kingdom of Morocco
Oulaiech Mohamed
19 Rue de Nador, Meknes
PHONE/FAX: (212) 05 514700

Kuwait
Kasim Demir
P.O. Box 8300,
Code No. 22053, Salmiya
PHONE: (965) 575 1274
FAX: (965) 575 5700

Kyrgyz Republic
An Innokentiy Nikolaevich
National Federation Karate-Do
Shotokan International Kyrgyz
Republic
720044,Kyrgyz Republic,
Bishkek,Str.Suhomlinova,52-A

PHONE: (996) 312 55 25 34 /
(996) 312 48 55 26
FAX: (996) 312 55 25 33
E-MAIL: ervial@elcat.kg

Kuwait
Mohammed AL Rashidi
Karate-Do Club of Kuwait
P.O. Box 48177, Sabahiya
PHONE: (965) 371 7743
FAX: (965) 572 2255
E-MAIL: alhadi007@hotmail.com

Lithuania
Alexander Matyushevskiy
Minijos 130 B-1, 5804 Klaipeda
PHONE: (370) 0126 275832
FAX: (370) 06 322545

Macau
Andre Avelino Antonio
Associacao De Karate-Do Obukan
P.O. Box No. 420, Macau
PHONE: (853) 304922, 307561
FAX: (853) 338261, 593839,
483146 (OFFICE)

Macedonia
M.D. Slave Pashoski, Dr.
St. Partizanska br. 155/2-12,
91000 Skopje
PHONE: (389) 91 361122
FAX: (389) 91 363072

Madagascar
Eve Lyne
5 Rue Ratsimilaho,
P.O. Box 13, Antananarivo 101
FAX: (261) 20 223 3986 /
(261) 20 222 2835
E-MAIL: photoram@dts.mg /
bonnetfils@simicro.mg

Ratafika Adolphe
SKI Madagascar
P.O. Box 605, Antananarivo 101

Malaysia
Dato' Zulkipli B. Mat Nor
Persatuan Karate-Do Police Diraja
Malaysia
D/A, Pejabat Latiham Police,
Jalan Semapak 54100,
Kuala Lumpur
FAX: (60) 03 235 6085 /
(60) 03 294 7950 (ATTN OSMAN)

Johnny Khoo
197 Magazine Road,
Penang 10300
PHONE: (60) 04 261 3949 /
(60) 03 651 6619 /
(60) 03 651 6621
FAX: (60) 04 263 6921 /
(60) 03 651 1159 /
(60) 04 899 2320

M & Irene Tiru
20, Jalan Teluki 2, Bukit Sentosa,
48300 Rawang, Selangor
PHONE: (60) 3 6021 3830

Paul John Chin
P.O. Box 10606,
88806 Kota Kinabalu, Sabah
PHONE: (60) 088 56733

Malta
Carmel Mifsud
Carina Schembri Street,
Hamrun HMR 02
PHONE: (356) 239801
FAX: (356) 244690

Mexico
Hiroshi Ishikawa
SKIF Mexico
Bosques de Lago #66 Fracc.
La Herradura C.P. 52760,
Edo. de Mexico
PHONE: (52) 5 589 1821 /
(52) 614 414 92 27
FAX: (52) 5 589 1821
E-MAIL: skifmexico@hotmail.com

Gabriel Garcia
SKIF Mexico
C. Laguna de Mexicanos 3512,
San Felipe,5a.Etapa,CP 31219,
Chihuahua,Chih, Mexico
PHONE: 52-(614) 414 9227
E-MAIL: skifmexico@hotmail.com

Myanmar
Ohn Win
No. 51, Nguwa Road,
Ahlone Township, Yangon
PHONE: (95) 01 579919

Namibia
Johan Roets
SKIF Namibia
P.O. Box 1016,
Otjiwarongo

Negara Burunei Darussalam
PG. Sabri
No. 3 SPG 41 Lot 15773,
KG, Kiarong,
Bandar Seri Begawan
PHONE: (673) 383641

Nepal
Nivas G. Vaidya
SKI Nepal, Chief Instructor
L.P.O. Box 74, Mandhawan,
Lalitpur
PHONE: (977) 01 521353 /
(977) 01 535827
FAX: (977) 01 540679
E-MAIL: vaidya@umn.mos.com.np

Om Narayan Shrestha
Nepal Eco Tours (P.) Ltd.
G.P.O. Box 12398,
Osho Bhawan 3/Fl,
Clock Tower, Kamaladi,
Kathmandu
PHONE: (977) 01 225197 /
(977) 01 220055 /
(977) 01 243106
FAX: (977) 01 220054
E-MAIL: eco@mos.com.np

Netherland
Biagio Ridolfo
SKI Holland
Harmoniepolder 5
5235 TG's-Hertogenbosch,
Holland
PHONE/FAX: (31) 73 612 2721
E-MAIL: ski-holland@planet.nl

G. Beerends
SKI Netherland
Prof. Kam. Onneslaan 137a,
3112 Ve Schiedam
PHONE/FAX: (31) 10 4737865

New Caledonia
Fourn Justin
P.O. Box 1054,
Noumea
PHONE: (687) 263696
FAX: (687) 263684

New Zealand
Goran Glucina
16 Batkin Road,
New Windsor, Auckland 1007
PHONE: (64) 09 828 8310 /
(64) 025 284 7126
FAX: (64) 09 828 8310

Paul B. J. Wang M.D.
23 Wadekey Road,
Ilam, Christchurch 8004
PHONE: (64) 03 358 0702
FAX: (64) 03 358 0579

Stephen Hpa
15 rembrandt Avenue,
Tawa, Wellington 6006
PHONE: (64) 04 232 0215

Nicaragua
Esaul Loza
SKIF Nicaragua
Apartado Postal,
No 2496832 Managua,
PHONE/FAX: (505) 2496832
E-MAIL: elozap@yahoo.com

Francisco Esteves
Embajada de Espana
Apdo. 10150-1000, San Jose
PHONE: (506) 289 47798
FAX: (506) 222 4180
E-MAIL: franadri@sol.racsa.cr.oo

Niger
Alhaji Hamidou Abdou
P.O. Box 2286, Niamey
PHONE: (227) 740497 Niamey

Nigeria
Emmanuel Metu
SKI Nigeria, Technical
IMO State Sports Council,
Owerri

Folarunsho Alaran
SKI Nigeria, Financial
P.O. Box 22806,
U.1. Post Office, Ibadan,

Goby G.O. Shina
P.O. Box 22806,
University of Ibadan,
Oyo State, BP 06-591 Cotonou,
Benin

Onyekachi Omenuko
SKI Nigeria, Administrative
61 Wogu Street,
Port Harcourt,

Pakistan
Mahmood Naveed
78-A Garden Block,
New Garden Town, Lahore,
PHONE: (92) 042 863198
FAX: (92) 042 5836468

Palestina
Dirgham Jamal Khalil
P.O. Box 20898,
East Jerusalem, Via Israel
PHONE/FAX: (972) 02 279 6841

Panama
Juan Antonio de Leon
Via Italia,
Edif. Parque Mar, Planta Baja
PHONE: (507) 269 7253
FAX: (507) 223 7365

Ruben Fung
Asociacion Universitaria de
Karate-Do Panama
P.O. Box 6-3465 E1 Dorado,
Panama Rep. of Panama
PHONE: (507) 617 4227
FAX: (507) 236 2460
E-MAIL: rfch@hotmail.com /
rfch@sinfo.net

Peru
Moron A Marcos
SKIF-Peru
Calle Brahms 201,
San Borja, Lima 41
PHONE: (51) 1 476 2893 /
(51) 1 475 5885
FAX: (51) 1 476 2893 (HOME)
E-MAIL: skifperu@terra.com.pe

Philippines
Crispino P. Reyes
SKI Philippines
c/o Central Colleges of the
Philippines
52 Aurora Blvd, Quezon City,
Metro Manila
PHONE: (63) 02 715 5170 /
(63) 02 716 0706
FAX: (63) 02 713 3361 /
(63) 02 715 0846
E-MAIL: breyes58@webquest.com

Portugal
Aguas Mario Albert
S.K.I. Portugal
Rua de Fez 1219, 4150-333 Porto
PHONE: (351) 22 618 8782 /
(351) 96 523 7829
FAX: (351) 22 537 1029
E-MAIL: maa@netcabo.pt

Reunion
Fuma Alix/Sudel
Daimonji Dojo
1 Bis, Rampes De Saint Francois,
97400, Saint-Denis

PHONE: (262) 302912
FAX: (262) 306795

Romania
Tetu Gheorghe
str. Castanului, bl. 62,
sc. B, ap.11, Fagaras 2300

Constantin Luca
SKI Romania, President
Federatia Romana S.K.I.
str. T. Pertea, bl. 6/B/4,
Brasov, Fagaras 2300
PHONE: (40) 268 211 583
FAX: (40) 68 215611, 211418,
150714
E-MAIL: nitramonia@nitramonia.ro

Matei Sategeran
SKI Romania, General Secretary
str. Castanului, bl. 62. sc. B,
ap.11, Fagars 2300
PHONE: (40) 68 218773 /
(40) 68 212774
FAX: (40) 68 212774

Russia
Alexander Maiboroda
1 Mostowaia Street, Chita
PHONE: (7) 302 223 5975
FAX: (7) 302 226 3704

Alexandr Alelekov
P.O. Box 164,
Nizhny Novgorod 603137
PHONE: (7) 8312 317641 /
(7) 8312 476728 (HOME)
FAX: (7) 8312 380188
E-MAIL: alelelkov@bereg.nnov.su

Kim Den Tkhe
172 Lenina Street,
Yuzhno-Sakhalinsk 693000
PHONE: (7) 4242 741331
FAX: (7) 4242 741209
INTERN. FAX: 504 41 62009

Ramzin Alexsandr
Novozhilova 7,
Vladivostock 690011
PHONE: (7) 4232 232246 /
(7) 4232 227244 /
(7) 4232 520277
FAX: (7) 4232 264925 /
(7) 4232 520277 (HOME)

Rwanda
Kambanda Callixte
Rwandan Karate Federation
B.P. 4793-Kigali

PHONE: (250) 08505364
E-MAIL: k_callixte@hotmail.com

Saint Lucia
Oliver Lawrence
St. Lucia Bushido Shotokan
Karate-Do Academy
c/o Radio St. Lucia
P.O. Box 660, Castries
PHONE: (1) 758 452 2337 /
(1) 758 452 4038 (HOME)
FAX: (1) 758 452 4038

Singapore
Michael Wong Hong Teng
Block 405, #18-35,
Pandan Gardens 600405
PHONE/FAX: (65) 01 548346

Slovenia
Ivan Ceruc
Solska Ulica 16a,
2342 Ruse (Maribor)
PHONE: (386) 62 663031, 319138
FAX: (386) 62 31582

South Africa
P. Sonny Pillay
Shotokan Karate International S.A.
P.O. Box 2272, Durban 4000
PHONE: (27) 31 563 2994
E-MAIL: sonnya@saol.com

Spain
Enrique Tendero
Shotokan Karate-Do International
Espana
Ciudad de Martos,
4, 45400 Mora, Toledo
PHONE: (34) 925 341816
E-MAIL: etendero@wanadoo.es

Jesus Fernandez Martinez
KunKyu Kai Dojo
Julian Romea No. 5,
2A, 28003 Madrid
FAX: (34) 91 559 1669
E-MAIL: jesusf@petrabax.net

Sri Lanka
Bonnie Roberts
204/1 De Seram Place
Colombo 10
PHONE: (94) 01 695926
FAX: (94) 01 447308

J. Y. Indre De Silva
Chathura Karate Association
No. 22, Laxapana Mawatha,
Jayanthipura, Battaramulla
PHONE: (94) 01 562892

Sultanate Oman
Farid M. Al-Shehebi
P.O. Box 18,
MAF, PC116
PHONE: (968) 678572 /
(968) 607696 (HOME)
FAX: (968) 678579

Sweden
Bebinno Akyol
Norra Parkgatan 25,
561 34 Huskvarna
PHONE: (46) 3 614 2917
FAX: (46) 3 612 0539, 671 4313

Yoshi Yukawa
Kungsholmsgatan 30,
112 27 Stockholm
PHONE: (46) 8 653 4575

Switzerland
Gitte Bjorn
SKI Switzerland, Secretary
Unterdorfstr. 8,
CH-5213 Villnacherm
PHONE: (41) 62 887 6338 /
(41) 56 442 5514 (HOME)
FAX: (41) 62 887 6780 /
(41) 56 442 5514 (HOME)

Rikuta Koga
SKI Switzerland, Chief Instructor
Via Varesi 54, 6600 Locarno
PHONE: (41) 91 751 3813 /
(41) 79 444 4903 (MOBILE)
FAX: (41) 91 752 2913

Taiwan
Li Ping Chu
Taiwan Karate Association, ROC,
Director
P.O. Box 117-781,
TaiPei Post Office, TaiPei,
PHONE: (886) 02 2702 9524
FAX: (886) 02 2705 9424
E-MAIL: tkftka@hotmail.com

Togo
Aniaku Peter
BP 12104, Tome
PHONE: (228) 00228 221891

Trinidad and Tobago
Mason, Ralph-Neville
S.K.I.F.T.T
5 Sanora Park, Point Cumara,
Caribbean, W.I.
PHONE/FAX: (1) 868 637 5307
E-MAIL: skiftt@tstt.net.tt

Ukraine
Sergey A. Denisenko
Ukrainian Shotokan Karate-Do
Federation
Post Box 1079, 244030, Sumy
PHONE: (380) 0542 276875
FAX: (380) 0542 276875 /
(380) 0542 258231

United Arab Emirates
Najjar M. Sameer
SKI-UAE
P.O. Box 1565, Ajman
PHONE: (971) 06 7446441
FAX: (971) 06 7446998
E-MAIL: Skiuae@emirates.net.ae

Mahmoud Tillawi
P.O. Box 44305, Abu Dhabi
PHONE: (971) 26 673840 /
(971) 506 424983
FAX: (971) 26 673840

Tristan Hernandez
P.O. Box 62090, Dubai
PHONE: (971) 04 643918

U.K.
Shinji Akita
30 Aplin Way, Isleworth,
Middlesex, TW7 4RJ
PHONE: (44) 20 8232 8785
FAX: (44) 20 8568 4070

Chris Chapman, Dr.
SKIEF, General Secretary
4 Turnberry Close, Bramcote
Grange, Chilwell Lane, Bramcote,
Nottingham NG9 3LX
PHONE: (44) 115 9176326
FAX: (44) 115 9594599
E-MAIL: chris@cbcboots.demon.co.
uk

James A. Hardie
4 Ratray Road, Peterhead,
Aberdeenshire, Scotland

Jim Palmer
19 Bohun Court, Wallance Park,
Stirling FK7 7UT, Scotland
PHONE: (44) 1786 815395 /
(44) 0585 437463 (MOBILE)
FAX: (44) 1786 473072
E-MAIL: jimpalmer@skif.freeserve.
co.uk

John Wise
172 Sussex Road, North Harrow,
Middlesex HA1 4NQ
PHONE: (44) 181 863 3546
FAX: (44) 181 426 0252

Roger Carpenter
SKKIF, Chairman
37 Alexandra Road, Windsor,
Berkshire, SL4 1HZ
PHONE: (44) 1753 621152
FAX: (44) 1753 858084
E-MAIL: roger@walnutree55.freeserve.
co.uk

Shiro Asano
SKIEF, Chief Instructor
421 Westdale Lane, Mapperley,
Nottingham NG3 6DH
PHONE: (44) 1159 608988
FAX: (44) 1159 030659

Uruguay
Carlos Pazos Riera
Avda. Dr. Enrique Legrand 5163,
Montevideo
PHONE: (598) 2 2090214, 2099395
E-MAIL: pazos@multi.com.uy

USA
Masaharu Sakimukai
P.O. Box 56953,
Jacksonville, FL 32241

Toshihiro Oshiro
917 Main Street,
Redwood City, CA 94063
PHONE: (1) 650 364 7653
FAX: (1) 650 364 1338

Victor Takemori
Wing (Hawaii) Inc.
1750 Komo Mai Drive, Pearl City,
Hawaii 96782
PHONE/FAX: (1) 808 455 9844

Charles Macolino
Jerry DiCanio
Long Island Shotokan
400 Hempstead Tpke,

W. Hempstead, NY 11552
PHONE: (1) 516 538 7382
FAX: (1) 516 538 0786
E-MAIL: LI_shotokan@aol.com

Albert Mallari Jr.
1421 Silver Avenue,
San Francisco, CA 94134
PHONE: (1) 415 468 2960

Almer Mallari
25 Gambier Street,
San Francisco, CA 94134
PHONE: (1) 415 239 4579

Benjamin Balanay
SKIF Konna-Hawaii Branch
P.O. Box 474, Capy. Cook,
Kona, Hawaii 96704
PHONE: (1) 808 323 3350

Bijan Soleimani
1563 Solano Avenue,
Ste 366, Berkeley, CA 94707
PHONE: (1) 510 559 8846
FAX: (1) 510 644 8267 /
(1) 510 549 0216

Brian R. Fey
Shotokan Karate-Do of Japan
Federation
P.O. Box 1843, Pinellas Park,
FLA., 34664-1843
PHONE: (1) 727 546 4844
E-MAIL: Pine_Waves@webtv.net

Bruce C. Barker
RR1, Box 2870 Dixmont,
Maine 04932

Charles E. Lee
239 Lyons Avenue,
Newark, NY 07112
PHONE: (1) 973 926 1422

Charles S. Baker
6844 Broadway Terrace,
Oakland, CA 94611
[SHOP]
1533 Polk Street, San Francisco, CA
PHONE: (1) 510 595 1255 /
(1) 415 775 2935

Clifford Sasano
Kaumakapili Dojo
c/o Robert Nishimura
916-A 10th Avenue, Honululu,
Hawaii 96816
PHONE: (1) 808 734 1387

Daniel T. Clinkscales
Danha Kai Dojo
104-38 164 Street, Jamaica,
NY 11433
PHONE: (1) 917 449 2897

Dennis R. Cuizon
2405 Anihinihi Street,
Pearl City, Hawaii 96782

Dennis T. Loebs
Pacific Coast Shotokan
11954 Inglewood Avenue,
Hawthorne, CA 90250
PHONE: (1) 213 679 3156 /
(1) 310 370 3921

Francis Fong
SKIUSA, President
3425 Ala Ilima Street,
Honolulu, Hawaii 96818-2332
PHONE: (1) 808 839 7864

Sidney Jiro Kanno
SKIF Konna-Hawaii Branch
P.O. Box 492, Kealakekua,
Kona, Hawaii 96750
PHONE: (1) 808 329 2809

George Lam
Shotokan Karate-Do Institute of
Kapolei
P.O. Box 700123,
Kapolei, Hawaii 96709
PHONE/FAX: (1) 808 674 6699

Glen Kennedy
Eastern Maine School of Self-
Defense
RR1 Box 3650, Levant, ME 04456
PHONE: (1) 207 884 3096

Glenn Stoddard
5703 Glenway Street,
McFarland, WI 53558
PHONE: (1) 608 838 6553 /
(1) 256 1003 (HOME)
FAX: (1) 608 256 0933

Glenna Burleson
P.O. Box 120904,
New Brighton, MW 55112
PHONE: (1) 651 631 2370
FAX: (1) 651 631 2379, 631 9634,
224 3345
E-MAIL: skifusa@aol.com

Hiroyasu Fujishima
The Calif. State University of
Northridge,
Depart. of Kinesiology & Phisical
Education, 18111 Nordhoff Street,
Northridge, CA 91330
PHONE: (1) 818 677 3205
FAX: (1) 818 677 3207

James P. Shea
72 Colland Green,
Colland, CT 06084
PHONE: (1) 860 896 1926
FAX: (1) 802 457 1392

Jay Castellano
85 Lester Avenue,
San Jose, CA 95125
PHONE: (1) 408 295 1226
(1) 408 238 2367

Joe Taylor
33 Park Avenue,
Monterey, CA 93940
PHONE: (1) 408 646 8088 /
(1) 392 0814 (HOME)

Jonathan Kwok
25115, S.E. 41 Drive,
Issaquah, WA 98029
PHONE/FAX: (1) 425 313 5671
E-MAIL: jonathan_kwok@yahoo.com

Lawrence Murley
9 Laurel Place #1, San Rafael, CA
PHONE: (1) 415 459 3954

Lisa B. Conesa
6504 Alta Vista Drive,
E1 Cerrito, CA 94530
PHONE: (1) 510 234 4881

Mark Richardson
258 Sunoi Street,
San Jose, CA 95126
PHONE: (1) 408 294 3838
FAX: (1) 408 294 5553

Mark Withrow
Pleasanton Shotokan Karate-Do
915-C, Main Street,
Pleasanton, CA 94566
PHONE: (1) 925 484 1954

Mary MacNab
1563 Solano Avenue,
Ste 463, Berkeley, CA94707
PHONE: (1) 510 559 8846

Masashi Yasuhiro
3338 Vincente Street,
San Francisco, CA 94116
PHONE: (1) 415 681 1435 /
(1) 650 583 0496
FAX: (1) 650 583 0497
E-MAIL: seibubos@gateway.net

Mike Cook
Maine Karate Association
P.O. Box 549, Framington,
Maine 04938
PHONE/FAX: (1) 207 778 0413
E-MAIL: gunner@somtel.com

Omayra Roman Munoz
P.O. Box 216, Aguas Buenas,
Puerto Rico 00703
PHONE: (1) 787 272 3153
FAX: (1) 787 732 8644

Patricia Milam
Tachi Dojo
Ernest Baldiviez
1533-B, So. Broadway,
Santa Maria, CA 93454
PHONE: (1) 805 925 2995
FAX: (1) 805 937 5269

Richard R. McGibbon Jr.
P.O. Box 828, Millinocket,
Maine 04462
PHONE: (1) 207 723 7988

Rick A. Montgomery
P.O. Box 2031, Medical Lake,
Washington 99022
PHONE: (1) 509 299 4804

Rigatcho Rey Hilario
350 E. Desert Inn Road,
Apt. 203, Las Vegas, Nevada 89109
PHONE: (1) 702 731 9702

Robert Halliburton
744 West Bullard, Fresno,
CA93704
PHONE: (1) 209 229 5104 /
(1) 209 432 5322 /
(1) 209 226 5121 (DOJO)
FAX: (1) 209 431 4301

Rufino Diaz
1514 Blueteal Drive,
Brandon, Florida 33511
PHONE: (1) 813 651 0370

Shadi Barazi
10611 Cedar Creek,
Houston, Texas 77057
PHONE: (1) 713 789 6465
E-MAIL: sbarazi@houston.rr.com

Sonny L. Kim
Japanese Karate-Do
11914 Montgomery Road,
Cinti-Ohio 45249
PHONE: (1) 513 697 8988

Steve D. Wong
Shotokan Karate-Do International
of Hawaii, Secretary
3375 Pakui Steet, Honolulu,
Hawaii 96816
PHONE: (1) 808 945 7882 /
(1) 800 734 8359 (HOME)
FAX: (1) 808 946 2563
E-MAIL: sdwpaw@juno.com /
mitsunaga001@hawaii.rr.com

Theresa Nichiporuk
Bronx Traditional Shotokan
Karate-Do
1626 Bronxdale Avenue,
BX, NY 10462
PHONE: (1) 718 822 1329
FAX: (1) 718 822 6498
E-MAIL: bronxshotokan@aol.com

Uzbekistan
Nurkhon Nafasov
National Karate Federation of
Uzbekistan
353, Korasaroy Street,
Tashkent, 700034
PHONE: (998) 712 487867 /
(998) 712 487565
FAX: (998) 71 1444838
E-MAIL: uzkarate@gimli.gimli.com /
Uzkarate@baht.gimli.com

Venezuela
Alejandro Castro B.
Kodokai Shotokan Karatedo Inter-
national
P.O. Box 40543, Ofi. Nva.
Granada, Caracas 1040
PHONE: (58) 2 633 2915
FAX: (58) 2 961 0066, 242 5342
E-MAIL: skif_kodokai@hotmail.com

Lic. Vicente Gonzalez Lopez
Union S.K.I. de Venezuela
Centro Commercial San Luis,
Planta Baja Local 19, Urb. San Luis,
E1 Cafetal, Caracas 1061

PHONE: (58) 2 986 9256
FAX: (58) 2 987 9325

Vietnam
Frank Gerke
Im Kierbusch 7, 53773 Hennef,
Germany
PHONE/FAX: (84) 49 2242 909741

Hoang Vinh Giang
Haoi Sports Department,
10, Trinh Hoai Duc Street, Hanoi
PHONE: (84) 42 64639, 32655
FAX: (84) 42 34457, 37474

Le Ba Truc
PC 26, 62 Nguyen Tat Thanh,
Buon Ma Thuot City, Daklak

Nguyen Van Ai
39 Banh Van Tran Street, Ward 7,
Tan Binh Dist, Ho Chi Minh City
PHONE: (84) 865 2350

Yugoslavia
Dot. Ziko G. Becanovic
Nusiceva 2,
24000 Subotica
PHONE: (381) 24 34903, 24 52116
FAX: (381) 24 52116